NO PILLS NO NEEDLES

To everyone who has or seeks to either reverse or prevent high blood pressure, diabetes and obesity
and
to all those who educate, influence and lead by example

NO PILLS NO NEEDLES

HOW TO REVERSE DIABETES AND HYPERTENSION BY FINDING OUT WHAT WORKS FOR YOU

Dr Eugene J Kongnyuy

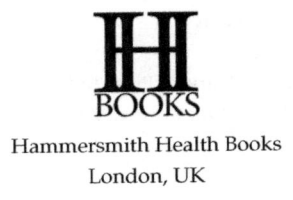

H BOOKS

Hammersmith Health Books
London, UK

First published in 2021 by Hammersmith Health Books – an imprint of
Hammersmith Books Limited
4/4A Bloomsbury Square, London WC1A 2RP, UK
www.hammersmithbooks.co.uk

© 2021, Eugene Kongnyuy

All rights reserved. No part of this publication may be reproduced, stored in any retrieval system or transmitted in any form or by any means, electronic, mechanical, photocopying, recording or otherwise, without the prior permission of the publisher and copyright holder.

The information contained in this book is for educational purposes only. It is the result of the study and the experience of the author. Whilst the information and advice offered are believed to be true and accurate at the time of going to press, neither the author nor the publisher can accept any legal responsibility or liability for any errors or omissions that may have been made or for any adverse effects which may occur as a result of following the recommendations given herein. Always consult a qualified medical practitioner if you have any concerns regarding your health.

Disclaimer
The views expressed herein are those of the author and do not necessarily reflect the views of UNFPA or the United Nations.

British Library Cataloguing in Publication Data: A CIP record of this book is available from the British Library.

Print ISBN 978-1-78161-192-0
Ebook ISBN 978-1-78161-193-7

Commissioning editor: Georgina Bentliff
Designed and typeset by: Evolution Design & Digital Ltd, Kent, UK
Cover design by: Madeline Meckiffe
Index: Dr Laurence Errington
Production: Deborah Wehner, Moatvale Press Ltd, UK
Printed and bound by: TJ Books Ltd, Cornwall, UK

Contents

About the Author   *vii*
Acknowledgements   *viii*

Introduction:
No pills, no needles   1

Chapter One:
Trial and error   5

Chapter Two:
Sick fat disease   19

Chapter Three:
Your diet – getting it right   29

Chapter Four:
Overweight and obesity   43

Chapter Five:
Intermittent fasting   63

Chapter Six:
Type 2 diabetes   79

Chapter Seven:
High blood pressure   97

Chapter Eight:
Exercise   107

Chapter Nine:
Drinking alcohol   119

Chapter Ten:
Smoking 129

Chapter Eleven:
Stress 143

Chapter Twelve:
Try, track and tell 157

Chapter Thirteen:
Changing your lifestyle 167

Chapter Fourteen:
A healthy living environment 175

Glossary of terms **183**
References **191**
Index **199**

About the Author

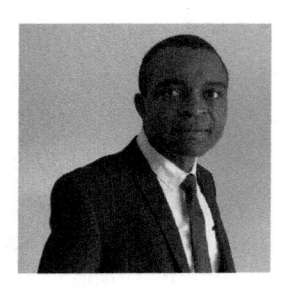

Dr Eugene J Kongnyuy, MD PhD, is a physician, researcher, educator and diplomat. He was born in Cameroon. After obtaining his medical degree, he moved to the United Kingdom for further studies. He is a Consultant Obstetrician and Gynaecologist and a global health expert with a PhD from Staffordshire University, UK. He was Clinical Lecturer in Sexual and Reproductive Health at the University of Liverpool before joining the United Nations. He has served with the United Nations Population Fund (UNFPA) since 2009 in several senior positions across many countries.

Dr Kongnyuy is known for his research and work in the area of women's health, particularly on high blood pressure during pregnancy, gestational diabetes, obesity and oestrogen-replacement therapy during menopause. He is also known for his ability to simplify complex concepts and connect with an audience through storytelling.

Acknowledgements

My journey with both diabetes and high blood pressure has been both distressing and gratifying. I thank the Almighty God for giving me his blessing and showing me the way to a natural but priceless solution that has enabled me to say 'goodbye to pills'. I sincerely acknowledge my wife, Yvette, who stood by me at all times during this journey and showed me the love and consolation that kept me inspired. This book is the fruit of her care, insights, encouragements and endorsements. It's her book!

To my kids Roy, Glen and Beri, I say, 'Thank you for being the source of my motivation and curiosity. You persuaded me to look at things from different perspectives. I'm proud of you.'

To my entire family, I lack words to express my gratitude and appreciation – I owe you so much! To my sister-in-law, Charlotte, you encouraged and supported me to step out of my comfort zone. I can't thank you enough.

Introduction

No pills, no needles

No Pills, No Needles *is a true life story. I took pills for high blood pressure and diabetes for several years. Through trial and error, I reversed both conditions and stopped taking medicines.*

When I was diagnosed with high blood pressure and type 2 diabetes, I was faced with two options. Either I took pills for the rest of my life or I figured out how to reverse the two conditions so that I could live healthily without medicines.

As a physician myself, I knew reversing both high blood pressure (also known as 'hypertension') and diabetes was almost impossible. I had been taught in medical school that both conditions were chronic diseases. By nature, they were incurable. In the past, I had told my patients with these two conditions that they had to take medications for the rest of their lives. I had counselled them to take these medicines to avoid complications that could be life-threatening.

Now, the patient was myself and my doctor had told me the same thing I had been telling my patients. I agreed with my doctor and started taking antidiabetic and antihypertensive pills, but while taking these medicines, I remained curious. There was a big question that I couldn't answer:

> *If high blood pressure and diabetes are caused by an unhealthy lifestyle, such as physical inactivity and poor eating habits, why should these conditions not be reversed if one switches to a healthy lifestyle?*

I decided that I would spend the rest of my life, if necessary, experimenting through trial and error to find an answer. I didn't follow any complicated research rules. I needn't have any funding for my research. I was the patient *and* the researcher. I didn't want to do anything complicated. My approach was based on my instinct as a doctor, with no specific rules to tie me down. Intuitively, based on my training as a scientist, I followed three simple steps for each change in lifestyle I trialed. I called these steps the '3Ts of trial and error'.

- Step 1: **T**ry (try out)
- Step 2: **T**rack (monitor)
- Step 3: **T**ell (know/recognise)

I 'try' something, I 'track' or monitor my blood pressure and blood sugar, and finally I 'tell', or know, whether or not it works.

I tried out many different things using these three steps. I tried out a range of dietary changes involving either inclusion or exclusion of specific food items or supplements. I tried different forms of physical activity and exercise. I tried different stress management techniques. I left no stone unturned.

In total, I conducted 70 trials over five years. Through these trials, I discovered what to do to stop taking antidiabetic and antihypertensive medicines. My blood pressure dropped to the normal range and my blood sugar also reversed to normal.

Introduction

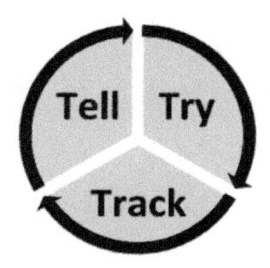

Figure 1: The 3 Ts of trial and error

This book is about my story, a true story of what I did to reverse diabetes and high blood pressure, and the lessons I learnt. Everyone is different. While my story may not be replicated by everyone, the lessons will work for many and the method can be used by all.

Chapter One

Trial and error

I conducted 70 trials on myself (self-experimenting) which helped me discover how to recover completely and stop taking medicines for high blood pressure and type 2 diabetes.

> **Lesson 1**
>
> High blood pressure and type 2 diabetes can be completely reversed, provided you adopt the appropriate lifestyle.

During one of my routine health checks, my doctor took my blood pressure and it was 150/100 mm Hg.

'Your blood pressure is high!' she told me. 'This may be due to white-coat hypertension. We need to confirm whether or not you really have high blood pressure. You will need to take your blood pressure at home every morning and evening for one week.' 'White coat hypertension' occurs when someone's blood pressure is high in the doctor's office or hospital (due to anxiety) but not at home or in other settings.

'Should I come back with the results in a week's time?' I asked.

'Yes, Tuesday next week at 10 am. I hope this is fine for you?' she replied.

I left the GP's surgery (general practitioner's office) in Salisbury, UK, feeling devastated. As a physician myself, I believed high blood pressure (or hypertension) had no cure. I had never seen a person cured of it. It was going to be tough. It would change the way I did things and my lifestyle forever. Worse still, I would end up with complications in my heart and kidneys, and might even have a stroke. The diagnosis of high blood pressure (BP) is not a death sentence, but it is close to that.

I went home and ensured that I took my BP every morning and evening for a week. It remained high throughout the week. I tried to take a rest during the day and started doing exercise. That week was a terrible week in my life because I was coming to terms with the fact that I had high blood pressure. But, why me? I was still young – at 39, life had hardly started.

My family was there for me. My wife, Yvette, consoled me, telling me that all would be fine. She asked me to slow down my pace of work and get more rest. She searched online and found that reducing salt intake could reduce blood pressure. That day she cooked and didn't add any salt to the food. Although, it wasn't tasty without salt, we both ate it - she also, although she could've added salt to her portion.

After a week, I went to see my GP and showed her my BP records. She took my BP again and it was high. Although the actual readings varied, all were consistently above 130/90 mm Hg. This was indicative of high BP – hypertension.

'Your blood pressure is 148/97 mm Hg. Let me take it again,' she said.

'Waaooh!' I tried to get control as my lower lip was trembling.

'The results of the lab tests that you did last week are out. Your blood sugar is high. All the other tests are normal,' she added.

'Does it mean I've got diabetes?' I asked, anticipating the worst case scenario.

'No, we don't know yet. You will need to redo the fasting blood sugar. In addition, you will need to do the glycated

Chapter One

haemoglobin test. We can only confirm diabetes if your glycated haemoglobin is high,' she explained. Glycated haemoglobin is a measure of the average blood sugar level over the previous three months.

My glycated haemoglobin came back high.

My doctor gave me a month to try first-line treatment consisting of lifestyle changes, particularly diet and exercise. She advised me to lose weight and do more exercise. If my BP and blood sugar didn't normalise after one month, I was going to be put on pills for both high blood pressure and diabetes. I would have to take the medicines for the rest of my life. That was particularly scary to me. Out of the blue, my health had worsened sharply. I had moved from being hale and hearty to being sickly with two incurable illnesses.

During the month my GP had given me, I was more determined than ever to do everything I could to reverse the two dangerous conditions. I hated exercise. I had hated exercise since childhood. But, this was not the moment to think about whether or not I liked it. I had no alternative but to be more physically active. Every day, I went to the park to exercise. I preferred walking to running. My daughter, Beri, loved going to the park and so she would go with me. While she played on the swings, seesaws, playhouses, slides, chin-up bars and spring riders, I walked or ran round the park. I forced myself to exercise until I was tired and couldn't continue. I did at least 30 minutes of exercise every day for a month. Most of the time during exercise I was walking.

With regard to dieting, I reduced my salt intake and tried to reduce my total calorie intake. I avoided unhealthy foods, such as sugary drinks, white bread, and cookies, and made sure I ate fruit and vegetables. Within a month I lost one kilogram in weight, but my BP didn't reduce.

The 'body mass index', or BMI, is used to determine whether someone is underweight, normal, overweight or obese. It is calculated as body weight (in kilos) divided by the square of the person's height (in metres). For adults, normal BMI is within the range 18.5 to 24.9. My doctor told me my BMI was 26.1, meaning I was overweight. Despite the efforts made over a month, my BMI changed just minimally. This was very discouraging. I recalled my lectures at medical school. We were told high blood pressure and diabetes were chronic diseases because they were incurable. I therefore concluded that irrespective of how much exercise and dieting I did, there wasn't going to be a solution without medicines.

At the end of the month, I returned to my GP to make the final decision whether or not to be put on pills. That morning, I did some intensive exercise with the hope that it could change my BP and diabetic status. It didn't. When I met my GP, she confirmed that my BP had remained high and that lifestyle change was not a suitable treatment for me. To lower my BP she put me on the 'ACE inhibitor' ramipril, 5 mg two times a day. She also prescribed metformin, an antidiabetic drug, 500 mg twice a day. She asked me to come back for follow-up in one month.

I was shocked. Within a month, I had been diagnosed with two deadly diseases. Diabetes in particular was frightening. Its complications are many and life-threatening and, when untreated, can lead to severe complications in almost all organs of the body, including the kidneys, eyes, brain, liver, feet and hands. My worries weren't just about taking pills. I was more concerned about the likely complications of both high blood pressure and diabetes.

Thirty trials for reversing diabetes

While taking pills, my blood sugar level remained borderline, between the upper end of normal and abnormal, fluctuating between the two. When I increased exercise and was careful with my diet while taking medicine, my blood sugar was normal, but when I relaxed my exercise regime and diet, it slipped into the abnormal range. My life changed with the diagnosis of type 2 diabetes: I resolved to take my antidiabetic medicine regularly, to walk for at least 30 minutes per day, and to avoid sugars and sweet drinks.

When my blood sugar was high, I urinated more frequently. Even without a test, I could sense when it was abnormally high. I bought a diabetes testing kit. I used it to monitor my blood sugar level. I found it rose to abnormal levels if I didn't stick to my diet, didn't do enough exercise and/or didn't take my medicines. I concluded that I had to take the medicine, do exercise and stick to my diet to keep diabetes under control. I would have to do this for the rest of my life.

Inwardly, I believed that there was a cure for diabetes. 'One day someone will discover it,' I told myself. But why wait for someone else to do it? As a physician and researcher, I had the right skill-set to conduct this type of research. So, I decided, I was going to conduct research on diabetes. My objective was to find a cure that would allow me and others to stop taking antidiabetic medicines. 'No pills, no needles' was my ultimate aim.

I decided not to follow any complicated research procedures. I didn't write any study protocol. I didn't look for any research grants. I chose to use myself as the subject for my research. I knew this was risky because if diabetes was not well controlled, I could end up with the complications I've already mentioned. I understood the risk I was taking. I was fully prepared. I decided not to stop taking antidiabetic medication during the trials, until I found something that was almost as effective as the medicine itself.

I chose myself as a subject for experimentation for many reasons. First, I didn't need my research to be approved by any ethical research committee. Secondly, by using myself for the experiment, it meant I would never be without a patient to study; I would be there at any time for the experiment. Thirdly, using myself also had the added advantage that the study participant remained the same for all trials (myself); what changed were the different interventions that I trialed. Fourthly, the trials would be faster since I could switch immediately from a failed trial to a new one without a break. Finally, it was an opportunity for me to use trial and error free of the strict rules of modern research. The drawback of the research was that it had only one participant. However, it didn't really matter. 'If I find a cure for myself, it should certainly work for millions of other people,' I told myself.

What I did was not completely new. Several scientists and doctors have experimented on themselves. I simply joined a long tradition of self-experimentation in science and medicine, with some notable examples listed in Table 1.

In the end, I conducted 30 trials on my diabetes over two years. On average, each took roughly four weeks. The trials were carried out either singly or in combinations. They included:

180 minutes of walking per week	no cow's milk
420 minutes of walking per week	gluten-free diet
meditation	avocados
sugar-free diet	nuts
leafy greens	whole grains
diet free of refined carbohydrates	raisins
limiting saturated fats	aloe vera
weight loss through calorie restriction	broccoli
more fruit	okra
higher-fibre starchy foods	ginseng
cinnamon	no alcohol
supplementation with chromium, zinc, calcium, magnesium, vitamin C, vitamin B complex, multivitamins	ginger

Chapter One

Table 1: Doctors and scientists who have experimented on themselves (not without considerable risk)

Scientist	Self-experiment
Sir Isaac Newton	Newton was studying optics and had a problem because some people saw strange coloured spots in front of their eyes. In order to determine whether the colours were caused by the eye, he conducted an experiment on himself by sticking a sewing needle between his eyelid and his eye. He documented that light and dark coloured spots appeared when he moved the needle but disappeared when he kept it still.
Sir Humphry Davy	Sir Humphrey Davy was a chemist who conducted an experiment on himself to find out what happens if you inhale strange fumes from chemical substances. His self-experiment led to the discovery of nitrous oxide or 'laughing gas' which is still used today as a sedative agent during surgery.
Jesse Lazear	Jesse Lazear was an epidemiologist who wanted to determine the cause of yellow fever. He suspected that a mosquito bite transmitted this dissease and to prove this he got himself bitten by an infected by mosquito. He contracted yellow fever and died.
Albert Hofman	Albert Hofman was a chemist who studied lysergic acid diethylamide (LSD) through self-experiment. He synthesised, ingested and learned about the hallucinatory effects of the drug.
Barry Marshall	In an effort to convince doctors that gastric ulcer was caused by a bacterium, *Helicobacter pylori*, Barry Marshall took some *H. pylori* from the gut of an ailing patient, stirred it into a broth and drank it. He then developed gastritis, the precursor of an ulcer. He biopsied his own gut and cultured *H. pylori* proving that bacterial infection was the cause of ulcers.

Each dietary trial generally involved adding one or more dietary item to my usual diet for a period of three to four weeks. However, when the trial involved eating calorie-rich foods, part of my regular calorie intake was replaced to avoid increasing overall calorie intake.

Each trial followed three simple steps based on my intuition as a trained doctor and researcher. I called them the 3Ts of trial and error – Try, Track, and Tell. I try something, I 'track', or monitor, my blood pressure and blood sugar, and finally I 'tell' whether or not it is effective. If it is ineffective, I try out something different.

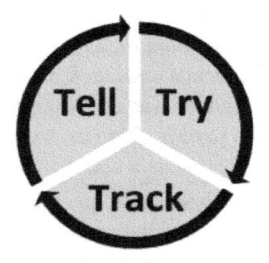

Figure 2: The 3Ts of trial and error

The results of the first 29 trials were discouraging. In almost two years, I wasn't able to find a cure for diabetes. None of the trials reduced my blood sugar significantly to allow me to stop antidiabetic medicine. My objective of saying goodbye to pills seemed elusive.

By stopping eating lunch and snacks, I lost 10 kg of my weight and my blood sugar dropped to normal

However, there were two trials that looked promising – namely exercise and weight loss. I observed that if I stopped exercise completely, irrespective of what I did, my blood sugar would rise to abnormal levels. I also observed that losing a few

Chapter One

kilos of body weight had a significant effect on my blood sugar level. However, it was difficult to sustain the weight loss. Exercise alone had very little effect on weight loss. Most of the weight loss had to come from my diet. Reducing the total quantity of food intake was also difficult. I got very hungry and weak when I tried to reduce total food intake significantly.

With a clue to what might be the cure for diabetes, I decided to modify my weight loss technique. My 30th trial involved stopping eating lunch and snacks. The first week, it was extremely difficult because I was used to taking lunch. However, with strong willpower, I managed not to eat during the day despite the hunger and weakness. In the second week, I became used to spending my day without lunch and snacks and that continued. In three months, I then lost 10 kg of weight (that is, 12.5% of my weight). I felt healthier. My blood sugar went down to levels I had never seen before. This was a breakthrough discovery.

Following the weight loss, I decided to stop taking metformin. That was risky because blood sugar levels could spike, but I was ready to take the risk. I took my blood sugar daily at home. It remained normal for two weeks without metformin. At last, I had found the cure for diabetes.

After three months, I went to see my GP. She asked me to do the fasting blood sugar and glycated haemoglobin tests. Both were normal. She asked me to come back after three months to redo the same tests. Both tests were normal after three months. I continued my daily exercise and 'no lunch, no snacks' strategy.

By stopping having lunch and snacks, I reduced my total calorie intake (carbohydrates, fats and proteins) by about 50% per day and lost 12.5% of my weight. My weight remained stable after I'd lost that 10 kg (12.5%). I had reduced my carbohydrate intake significantly. My total fat intake per day was also reduced but not as much as carbohydrates. I also noticed that, I ate less at dinner despite the fact that I didn't take lunch. That was contrary to what I had initially thought. I had thought I would have the tendency to eat more at dinner because I had skipped my lunch. In fact, the volume of my stomach shrank when I stopped having lunch. I got full easily when I ate dinner. I decided that once I felt full, I would stop eating.

While I was excited about my discovery of a cure for diabetes, my wife was worried about my weight loss. I had to change all my shirts, suits and trousers because they were now too big for me. My fatty tissue had shrunk beneath my skin leaving my skin loose and dry.

'Are you sure you are normal?' my wife asked. 'You look frail and pale.'

'Yes, I am absolutely normal. I am feeling better with this new weight. This is the only way to control my diabetes,' I reassured her.

'We need to see the GP. I don't think it's normal,' she insisted.

'OK, no problem. I'll call the GP Surgery and book an appointment,' I accepted reluctantly.

We went together to the GP on the day of the appointment. My wife expressed her concerns about the weight loss and the doctor smiled. After measuring my weight and conducting a clinical examination, the doctor reassured my wife that my weight was absolutely normal, and even desirable. My BMI had dropped from 26.1 to 22.8. By losing weight, I had moved from being overweight to normal weight.

After a few months, with regular exercise, my loose skin tightened up and any sagging completely disappeared.

Seventy trials to reverse high blood pressure (BP)

Before I started antihypertensive medicine, my BP was about 150/100 mm Hg. With regular exercise and antihypertensive medication, it dropped to 130/90 mm Hg, which was borderline high. My doctor was worried about it remaining borderline and was thinking of changing my medication, but I convinced her to

Chapter One

give me more time to work on my weight and do more exercise.

My first 30 trials, as mentioned above, were used for *both* diabetes and high blood pressure. I assessed the effectiveness of each trial on both conditions. Hypertension, or high blood pressure, seemed to be more difficult to reverse. Of the 30 trials conducted on diabetes, none was effective enough for me to stop the antihypertensive pills.

While I initially thought diabetes would be more difficult to cure than high blood pressure, the reverse was true. Like diabetes, exercise and weight loss contributed to lowering my BP, but this improvement was insufficient to free me from the ramipril prescribed by my doctor. The 10 kg weight loss was useful but insufficient. With the weight loss, exercise and BP medication, my BP dropped from borderline to normal. However, the drop was not enough for me to stop taking BP medication. One time, I stopped the medicine and my BP rose into abnormal territory, so I concluded that the weight loss and physical exercise were good but insufficient.

I decided to continue with my trials. Over three years, I conducted 40 additional trials on BP. These included:

restricting salt intake	beetroot
cutting back on caffeine	beans
	egg whites
increasing potassium intake	tea
	calcium-rich foods
changing to low-fat dairy products	garlic
	deep breathing
dark chocolate	working less
apricots	listening to soothing music
oatmeal	changing my expectations
cauliflower	focusing on issues I had control over
spinach	
cocoa	relaxing more

berries	laughter
lean meats	60 minutes of walking per day
oily fish	90 minutes of walking per day
olive oil	120 minutes of walking per day
soy	60 minutes of jogging or running
tomatoes	per day
carrots	

They were tried either singly or in combinations. As for diabetes, each dietary trial generally involved adding one or more dietary item to my usual diet for a period of three to four weeks. However, when the trial involved eating calorie-rich foods, part of my regular calorie intake was replaced to avoid increasing overall calorie intake.

The trials had different effects on BP, ranging from no effect to small reductions. None led to a significant reduction in my BP. None was able to replace ramipril, my BP medicine.

One hour of working out per day for six months reduced my BP to the level I could stop my BP medicine

The results of all the 70 trials for BP were extremely discouraging. I had found a cure for my diabetes. I strongly believed there was one for high BP. After losing 10 kg, my BMI was down to normal. I was no longer overweight. Even with the weight loss, my BP was normal only when I combined exercise and pills. Further weight loss would be difficult to sustain and would raise more concerns from my family, especially my wife who didn't want to see me lose more weight.

I decided to continue with my 'no lunch, no snack' and one hour of jogging or running every day as this combination had yielded the best results.

Chapter One

After six months of working out for one hour each day, I had gained muscles. My calf muscles and biceps stood out visibly, showing that I was physically fitter. I enjoyed looking at the six-pack on my belly and taking selfies. I then decided to check my BP again (I had not been checking regularly as this was no longer a 'trial' as far as I was concerned) and to my great surprise it was very low, lower than any BP value I had recorded before.

One hour of workout (jogging and running) per day for six months had reduced my BP to the level at which I could stop my BP medicine. I had initially concluded that exercise (jogging and running) was ineffective simply because I had tried this only for one month. One month wasn't long enough for the exercise to have effect on my BP. While jogging and running for 60 minutes per day reversed my high BP in six months, walking 120 minutes per day for more than a year had proved ineffective.

I had continued jogging and running for six months because it was good to keep me fit and healthy in other ways. I had had no clue that it would reverse my high BP. And now, by accident, I had discovered that jogging and running could reduce my BP to a level at which I could stop BP medicine.

I stopped taking ramipril. I measured my BP daily to see what would happen. My BP remained within the normal range. I was free at last – free from pills.

My doctor was surprised. She checked my BP on a few occasions, and it remained normal. I could now start a new era of my life without thinking about pills or the future prospect of needles.

Conclusion

In total, I conducted 70 trials on high blood pressure. Of the 70 trials, jogging and running (which are considered moderate to vigorous aerobic exercise) had the biggest effect. I took a firm resolution to continue, for as long as I could, my 'no lunch, no snack' strategy for weight loss and one-hour workout (jogging and running) daily. These are the two things that helped me to stop antidiabetic and antihypertensive pills.

Following these successful trials, I have continued to try out new ideas, and to 'track' and 'tell'. Over time, I have understood more about preventing or reversing obesity, diabetes and high blood pressure. I have also come to discover easier ways to adopt good habits and get rid of bad ones.

The chapters that follow include the details of my experience and lessons learnt as to how to prevent or reverse obesity, hypertension and diabetes. I also show how my lessons and experience are backed by credible scientific evidence. The combination of obesity, high blood pressure and diabetes is called 'sick fat disease' (or 'metabolic syndrome'). This is caused by eating too much and moving too little.

Chapter Two

Sick fat disease

I was devastated when the doctor told me I was overweight, diabetic and hypertensive. That sparked the beginning of a long journey that turned my life around for the better.

> **Lesson 2**
>
> While the detection of potentially life-threatening conditions can be shocking, this can be the biggest wake-up call to change your lifestyle for the better.

The 2010 oil spill in the Gulf of Mexico was the worst in US history and is still one of the worst environmental disasters the world has seen. It led to the deaths of 11 oil-rig workers. Oil gushed into one of the earth's most diverse marine habitats killing millions of marine mammals, birds, fish and sea turtles. Interim measures, such as using chemicals to disperse the oil and floating booms to stop the oil from spreading, were used. However, the ultimate solution came when British Petroleum (BP) succeeded in capping the leakage.

The oil spill story may look extreme and irrelevant, but something analogous is occurring in our bodies, on a smaller scale, every day. The human body is a micro-planet. Oil provides a liquid fossil fuel (which comes from the sun, captured through photosynthesis) for our planet earth, while carbohydrates (or carbs) and fats provide fuel for our body. Excess carbs are converted to body fats. Fats are normally stored under the skin but excess fats spill over into vital organs of the body, such as the liver, kidneys, heart and brain. The overspill of fats to vital organs causes organ malfunction. This leads to obesity, high blood pressure and eventually type 2 diabetes. People who have diabetes are more likely to be obese and also more likely to have high blood pressure (hypertension). *'Sick fat disease' (also called 'metabolic syndrome' – introduced in the previous chapter)* is a name used to describe this malfunctioning, including obesity, hypertension and diabetes, caused by fat spill in the body.

Sick fat disease is caused by fat spill to internal body organs, which causes organ malfunction

I was overweight and had both high blood pressure and type 2 diabetes. This meant that I had sick fat disease. However, not everyone with sick fat disease will have obesity, high blood pressure *and* diabetes. This is because the damage caused by the fat spill is progressive.

You can remember the defining elements of this condition using **ABCD**:

A = Abdominal obesity
B = Blood pressure (high)
C = Cholesterol (high)
D = Diabetes (type 2)

With fat spill, large amounts of *'free fatty acids' (FFAs)* are released into the bloodstream. FFAs are the form in which fats leave the cells and are transported to another part of the body.

They reach the heart, brain and other organs, causing malfunction. The body declares a 'state of emergency' and releases 'riot police' called *cytokines* to restore order. Cytokines are proteins produced by defence (or immune) cells to regulate many body functions. The cytokines are bound to remain for as long as there is an emergency. If the state of emergency is prolonged, the prolonged presence of large amounts of cytokines in the blood instead of restoring order, makes things worse.

Cytokines and FFAs cause – guess what – high blood pressure, type 2 diabetes, and high cholesterol. Cytokines also cause inflammation and increase the risk of blood clot formation. Blood clots can block blood supply to vital organs and cause serious life-threatening conditions. When a blood clot blocks blood supply to the heart, this causes the life-threatening condition called heart attack.

*Cytokine*s are the body's 'police'. They are produced to regulate body functions and restore order when there is an emergency from within, as I have said. Like the police force on our streets, they take action to protect the body from disorders or imbalances in the internal environment, but when their presence is prolonged, their actions instead cause damage to the body. On the other hand, the antibodies are the 'soldiers' – they are produced to fight against foreign bodies such as viruses and bacteria that have invaded our bodies.

Abdominal obesity

Overeating can lead to overweight or obesity. Excess carbs or fat from overeating are subsequently converted and stored as fats. There are two main locations of fat storage in obesity: the lower body (hips and thighs) and upper body (belly/abdomen).

In lower-body obesity, the fat is located under the skin. This is a relatively harmless location for it to be stored. You can't determine how big your hips and thighs should be, but if you could, this is the place to store fat. Fat in the hips and thighs is located under the skin (subcutaneous), while fat in upper body obesity is located in internal visceral organs. Free fatty acids released by internal organs can easily find their way into the liver where it can influence lipid production including cholesterol. This is why those who are 'lucky' to have bigger hips and thighs (rather than a bigger abdomen) are less likely to develop sick fat disease. Lower-body obesity is protective against sick fat disease.[1]

The second location for the overspill of stored fats is the abdomen (belly) or upper body. Once the space in the lower body is full, fat storage spills into the vital organs in the abdomen. The bowel, liver and kidneys are flooded with fats. This causes organ malfunction. Consequently, people with big bellies are at a higher risk of sick fat disease. Excessive fat in the belly is called abdominal or upper-body obesity.

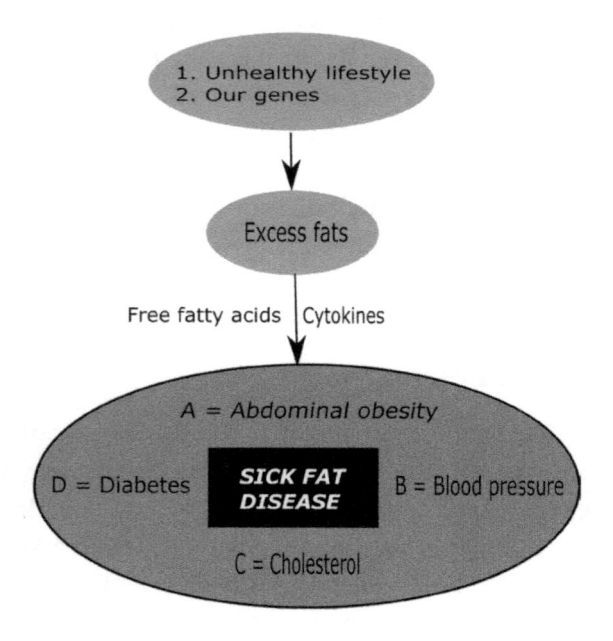

Figure 3: Unhealthy lifestyle causes sick fat disease

Blood pressure (high)

High levels of cytokines and free fatty acids in the blood trigger a chain of events that cause two things: sodium absorption by the kidneys and narrowing (contraction) of the blood vessels. These two things cause high blood pressure. The kidneys retain more sodium than usual that should normally have been excreted in urine as waste. Sodium increases the total blood volume and therefore blood pressure. When the blood vessels narrow (contract), this reduces the internal space available for the blood. This also causes our blood pressure to rise.

Cytokines and free fatty acids cause the kidneys to absorb sodium and the arteries to contract. Both actions raise blood pressure

The kidneys retain sodium and flush out potassium in the urine – in other words, they hang on to sodium at the expense of potassium. One way to flush out sodium from the body is to consume more potassium. Patients with high blood pressure are therefore often advised to restrict salt intake (table salt is sodium chloride) and increase potassium intake (bananas and oranges both contain lots of potassium).

Cholesterol (high)

Cholesterol (which is a type of fat and the precursor of many of our hormones) comes from the food we eat and from our liver. The liver doesn't only produce cholesterol; it also removes it from the body. However, high levels of cytokines and free fatty acids cause liver malfunction, which leads to high levels of cholesterol in the blood.

The liver is the body's 'chemical factory' and its malfunction causes serious damage to other body organs. One of the substances it produces is cholesterol. While cholesterol is often seen as our enemy, it is actually a crucial substance that performs numerous vital functions in the body. It is required for the synthesis of bile acids, which are essential for the absorption of fats. It is also needed for the synthesis of many hormones, such as testosterone, oestrogen, progesterone and cortisol. Together with sun exposure, cholesterol is needed for the production of vitamin D. It is found in cell membranes, where it provides structural support and may even serve as a protective antioxidant. It is essential for the normal functioning of the body's nervous (electrical) system where it plays a vital part in the transfer of electrical signals from one nerve fibre to another.

For decades, scientists have believed that excess amounts of low density lipoprotein (LDL) cholesterol cause atherosclerosis (buildup of plaque in artery walls), heart disease (a life-threatening condition where the blood supply to the heart is blocked) and stroke (a life-threatening condition where the blood supply to the brain is cut off). Fat, in the form of cholesterol, can build-up in the walls of arteries which over time forms plaque (atherosclerosis). Slowly, the blood vessels narrow and this impairs blood circulation and increases the risk of heart disease and stroke. This simplistic assumption that cholesterol directly and causally impacts atherogenesis (the process by which arterial plaques are formed) has been challenged in recent years.

A review of existing scientific literature failed to establish a direct cause-effect (causal) relationship between cholesterol and atherosclerosis/heart disease.[2] Another review concluded that inflammation, not cholesterol, is the cause of atherosclerosis which subsequently leads to heart disease.[3] These studies, and many others, suggest that cholesterol is a marker, rather than a cause, of atherosclerosis and heart disease. The explanation is that arteries are damaged by other factors, such as high blood pressure, inflammation and oxidative stress, and that cholesterol is used to repair the damage.

However, a large meta-analysis of randomised controlled trials involving 327,037 patients from 52 studies revealed that each 1 mmol/l reduction in LDL cholesterol was associated with a 19% reduction in the risk for major vascular events (stroke, heart attack, and death from a vascular disease). This suggests that LDL cholesterol may actually *contribute* to the development of atherosclerosis and heart disease.[4]

Based on the current evidence, it's clear that the role of cholesterol in the development of these problems is complex and not yet fully understood. A plausible explanation would be that cholesterol is not a direct cause, but a contributor to the causal chain (which involves many other factors/substances), increasing the risk of atherosclerosis and heart disease.

Cholesterol is carried through the bloodstream by proteins called 'lipoproteins' of which there are two types: LDL (low density lipoproteins) and HDL (high density lipoproteins). LDL has been called 'bad' cholesterol while HDL has been called 'good' cholesterol. The cholesterol ratio is the ratio of total cholesterol to HDL. The recommended ratio is between 3.5 and 1.[5] Excess LDL cholesterol is associated with an increased risk of heart disease and stroke. HDL cholesterol carries cholesterol from the body back to the liver and the liver removes it from the body. A high proportion of HDL cholesterol is therefore associated with a lower risk of heart disease and stroke. When your doctor asks for lab tests for cholesterol, s/he normally asks for levels of LDL, HDL and total cholesterol.

Diabetes

Type 2 diabetes is a condition characterised by high blood sugar. Insulin is a hormone produced by the pancreas to regulate blood sugar levels. For simplicity, look at insulin as the hormone that opens the doors of the body's cells for sugar to enter. When fats spill over into body organs, these doors are blocked so insulin can no longer open them. In response, the pancreas secretes more insulin, but the hormone is helpless because the doors are completely blocked by fats. The process is progressive such that initially the doors just don't open as wide as they should. Progressively, they become completely blocked. This situation is called 'insulin resistance'. The blood sugar level becomes high because sugar cannot find its way into the cells and insulin levels are also high because the pancreas keeps secreting more insulin in an effort to improve the situation.

Insulin is a 'key worker'. Hormones are the key workers that carry out essential functions without which we cannot stay alive. During the 2020 coronavirus pandemic, governments identified doctors, nurses, all healthcare workers, supermarket staff, care home workers, etc, as essential or 'key' workers. While everyone else was ordered to stay at home, the key workers continued to provide the essential services that people needed in order to survive. This is similar to what hormones do in the body.

Type 2 diabetes is caused by the failure of insulin to reduce blood sugar levels. Type 1 diabetes is caused by the failure of the pancreas to produce insulin

Type 2 diabetes occurs in sick fat disease due to insulin resistance. Type 1 diabetes on the other hand is the result of the pancreas failing to secrete insulin. In type 2 diabetes, insulin levels are high, while in type 1 diabetes they are low. Type 1 diabetes is not part of sick fat disease. It is reckoned that 95% of all cases of diabetes are type 2, while only 5% are type 1.

The best solution is prevention

Oil companies know the risks of oil spills and normally take action at two levels. The first is prevention. They identify the

Chapter Two

risks of such an event and take actions to mitigate those risks. The second is responding to an oil spill when it happens to reduce environmental, economic and human impact. There is general consensus that the best solution to an oil spill is prevention. This is equally true for human beings. The best solution to human 'fat spill disease' (or sick fat disease) is prevention.

To prevent or reverse sick fat disease, you need to adopt a healthy lifestyle. Use the SAFEST mnemonic to remember the lifestyle choices necessary to do this.

The 'safest' way to deal with sick fat disease is prevention so:

S = Smoking (stop)
A = Alcohol (moderate)
F = Food (eat healthily)
E = Exercise (do more)
S = Stress (avoid/reduce)
T = Treatment.

Smoking and stress increase our risk of sick fat disease. Drinking alcohol above recommended safe limits also increases the risk significantly. In the case of smoking, the risk is about 34% greater among active smokers. Extremely stressful life events, whether related to family, finance or work, increase the risk of obesity, high blood pressure and type 2 diabetes (see Chapter 6). Stressful life events increase the odd of sick fat disease by 13%.[6]

There are two main reasons people develop excess body fat: lifestyle and genetics. Our sedentary, overeating lifestyle is one of the major reasons sick fat disease has become a pandemic. We eat too much and move too little compared with decades ago. We eat far more carbs and fat than the body needs and yet we burn too little. We are not taking concrete measures to mitigate the risk of sick fat disease.

Our genes can make us more susceptible to sick fat disease. They affect our risk in two ways. Either we are born with a genetic predisposition or our genes adapt to a harsh environment, making us susceptible if this environment later improves. The latter is called 'epigenetics'. People who grow up in a harsh environment with an unstable food supply adapt to the conditions by maximising their storage of surplus food. If, later in life, conditions change and food becomes abundant, they are more predisposed to obesity. Their genes are already conditioned to conserving energy through body fat stores. This was first observed by James Neel, an American geneticist, in 1962. He called this the *'thrifty genotype hypothesis'*.[7]

Neel's observation is particularly important among people below the poverty line today. Some children who are dependent on adults on low incomes grow up not having enough food or only just enough. Once they reach adulthood, they may start working and having money of their own. They can now eat as much as they want. The change from a limited or controlled food environment to one of excess can lead to obesity.

Don't assume that you have obesity genes because your parents and siblings are obese. It may be due to the eating habits you have developed in the family. And if you truly have a genetic predisposition, you are not totally helpless. You may still achieve results by doing more than the average person – exercising more, paying more attention to your diet and putting in more effort to lose weight.

Chapter Three

Your diet – getting it right

In order to lose weight, I cut down my total food intake. My new diet didn't have the proper mixture of all the nutrients. As a result, I developed calcium deficiency.

> **Lesson 3**
>
> Efforts to lose weight can lead to an unbalanced diet; therefore, as you eat less to lose weight, make sure your diet remains balanced.

Delighted with my new fitness, I paid little attention when my nails gradually turned dry and brittle and my skin also slowly became dry. I didn't link these symptoms to a possible nutrient deficiency. To me, it wasn't something to worry about. 'These problems will probably go away soon,' I told myself.

The wake-up call came when one morning I woke up and felt severe pain in my neck. At that moment, I knew something was seriously wrong. As a physician, a thousand and one things that could cause the pain flew into my mind. In particular, I thought of muscle cramp or a 'slipped disc' (a condition where the soft tissue cushion between the bones in the spine pushes out). If it was muscle cramp, why were my muscles contracting? I had never felt such pain in my neck before and so I knew something was amiss.

I decided to go and see my doctor. After examination and laboratory tests, she told me that I didn't have enough calcium. I immediately recalled that when I had decided to lose weight, I had cut down my intake of everything, including dietary sources of calcium such as green leafy vegetables, dairy and alternatives. That was the cause of my calcium deficiency.

That was a big lesson for me. While reducing your food intake in order to lose weight, focus on reducing calorific foods (carbs, fats and proteins) which are the cause of weight gain. Make sure that you have adequate intake of dairy products and/or fruit and vegetables. Only reduce dairy, fruit and vegetables if you are consuming more than the recommended daily intake. Nutrient deficiencies can cause life-threatening problems. Calcium deficiency, for instance, can even cause high blood pressure.

This bitter experience reminded me to be careful about nutrition and, indeed, everyone should be. While there is a lot of information available on nutrition, the main problem is sorting out the facts from the myths and misleading claims by some food companies. I can sum up the most important dietary lessons into three points:

- Make a deliberate effort to eat healthily
- Be aware of what to eat more of and what to avoid
- National food guides have failed to halt the obesity pandemic.

Make a deliberate effort to eat healthily

To eat healthily, you must first understand what is a healthy, balanced diet. A balanced diet is one that gives your body the energy and nutrients it needs to work properly – what foods to eat in the right amounts.

Chapter Three

Processes such as thinking, pumping blood around the body and breathing require energy. Apart from breastmilk, there is no other single food that provides all the essential nutrients and energy that the body needs to stay healthy and function properly. There are therefore two dimensions to a balanced diet: quality and quantity. With regard to quality, we need to choose our daily food intake from the five food groups (UK Eatwell Guide):

- fruit and vegetables
- oils
- meat, fish, eggs, beans, pulses and other proteins
- dairy and alternatives
- starchy carbohydrates.

These are the foods that should be consumed in the right amounts.

After learning my bitter lesson, I now make sure that I get enough from each food group every day. My challenge is that national food guides remain controversial, differ between countries and are subject to change.

A balanced diet means healthy FOODS in the right amounts:

F = Fruit and vegetables
O = Oils
O = 'Ox' (beef and other types of meat), fish, eggs, beans, pulses and other proteins
D = Dairy and alternatives
S = Starchy carbohydrates

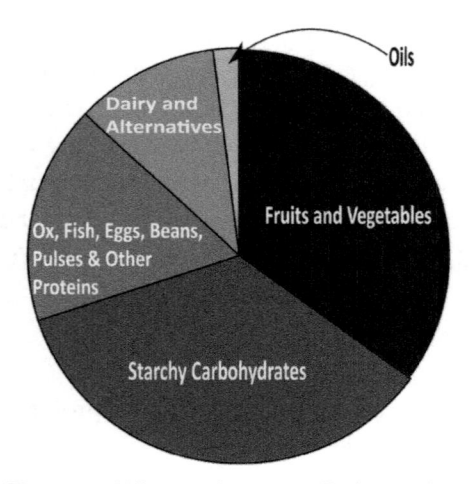

Figure 4: What makes up a 'balanced diet'

1. Fruit and vegetables

Fruit and vegetables should constitute about one-third of what we eat each day. They are a good source of fibre, vitamins and minerals. Eating a lot of fruit and vegetables can reduce the risk of obesity, heart disease, stroke and cancer. Beans and pulses fall into the fruit and vegetables group as well as the protein group. It's recommended that we consume at least five portions of a variety of fruit and vegetables per day.

If we eat more than one portion of beans and pulses, only one portion will count as fruit and vegetables because they don't contain the same combinations of vitamins, minerals and other nutrients as fruit and vegetables do. According to the UK *Eatwell Guide*, a portion of fruit and vegetables is:

- 80 g of fresh fruit and vegetables (about one medium-sized fruit, such as a banana, apple or pear) or
- 30 g of dried fruit (about a tablespoon) or
- 150 ml of unsweetened 100% fruit juice or
- 80 g of beans, peas and lentils.

Chapter Three

Fruit juice and/or smoothies should be limited to a total of 150 ml per day because of the sugar content.

Table 2: Balanced diet chart (*UK Eatwell Guide*)

Groups	What counts	Benefits	How much
Fruit and vegetables	• Fruit: banana, orange, grapefruit, pear, apple, strawberries, avocado, etc • Vegetables: spinach, sweetcorn, carrots, tomatoes, broccoli, lettuce, etc • Beans and pulses: beans, peas, lentils	Source of fibre, vitamins and minerals	5 portions of a variety of fruit and vegetables each day. This should be about 1/3 of what we eat each day.
Oils	• Vegetable oil, rapeseed oil, olive oil, sunflower oil, hemp oil, linseed oil	Source of essential fatty acids.	3 portions per day; required in small amounts. Make sure you eat a correct balance of omega 6 to omega 3 (3:1).
'Ox' (meat), fish, eggs, beans, pulses and other proteins	• Beans and pulses: beans, peas, lentils, chickpeas • Fish: oily fish, white fish, shellfish • Meat, poultry and game • Eggs • Nuts and peanut butter • Vegetarian alternatives: tofu, mycoprotein	Source of proteins, minerals, vitamins and fats	2 portions of fish per week (1 portion must be oily fish); not more than 70 g of red meat per day.

Groups	What counts	Benefits	How much
Dairy and alternatives	• Dairy: milk, yoghurt, cheese • Dairy alternatives: soya drink, soya yoghurt, oat milk, nut milk, rice milk	Source of protein, vitamins, calcium and iodine	3 portions per day
Starchy carbohydrates	• Rice, pasta, noodles, couscous, wheat, millet, sorghum, quinoa, cornmeal, oats, barley, rye • Bread and bread products • Potatoes and potato products • Yam, cassava, plantain.	Source of energy, fibre, vitamins and minerals	One third of total daily food intake.

For my breakfast, I normally have raisins (dried fruit), a piece of fruit (e.g. one apple), almonds, muesli, and dairy or alternatives (milk, yoghurt or alternatives) . This provides me with two portions of 'fruit and vegetables' (raisins and a piece of fruit) and two portions of dairy/alternatives . At dinner, I include the other three portions of fruit and vegetables in order to get the five per day recommended. I love beans because they are both 'fruit and vegetables' and 'protein'.

2. Oils

Oils are an essential part of a balanced diet and are required in small amounts. They provide us with essential fatty acids that can't be made by the body. They also help us absorb fat-soluble vitamins A, D, E and K. You should eat more of the polyunsaturated fats and less of the saturated fats.

Scientists have for long believed that saturated fat increases the risk of heart disease and stroke. However, a meta-analysis of 21 prospective cohort studies involving 347,747 participants followed up for 5 to 23 years showed that intake of saturated fat did not increase the risk heart disease and stroke.[8]

Another meta-analysis of randomised controlled trials, this time involving 56,000 participants from 15 studies, showed that cutting down on saturated fat led to a 17% reduction in the risk of cardiovascular disease (including heart disease and stroke). The review found that the health benefits arose from replacing saturated fats with polyunsaturated fat or starchy carbohydrates. It was found that the greater the decrease in saturated fat and the more total cholesterol was reduced, the greater the protection from heart disease and stroke. People who are currently healthy seem to benefit as much as people who are at risk of heart disease (diabetes, high blood pressure, high cholesterol) and people who have previously had heart disease or stroke. There was no difference in effect between women and men.[9]

Findings from these two meta-analyses described above suggest that it might well be the ratio of dietary polyunsaturated fat to saturated fat that determines the risk of cardiovascular disease, rather than saturated fat alone. Indeed, one study reported a reduced risk of cardiovascular disease when the ratio of polyunsaturated fat to saturated fat was greater or equal to 0.49.[10]

Fats have a high level of calories (energy) and therefore should be consumed in limited amounts. Common sources of saturated fat include red meat, whole milk and other whole-milk dairy foods, including cheese, and coconut oil. Unsaturated fats are fats that have one or more double bond(s) in their molecular structure and can be either polyunsaturated (with many double bonds) or monounsaturated (with a single double bond). Polyunsaturated fats are a source of omega 3 and 6, while monounsaturated fats are a source of omega 9. Common sources of monounsaturated fats are olive oil, peanut oil, canola oil, avocados and most nuts, as well as high-oleic safflower and sunflower oils. Dietary sources of omega 6 include nuts, pumpkin seeds, walnuts, hulled sesame seeds and most vegetable oils such as sunflower oil, linseed oil, hemp oil, safflower oil, corn oil and soybean oil. Dietary sources of omega 3 include oily fish (salmon, tuna, mackerel, herring, sardines), nuts and seeds (flaxseed, walnuts, chia seeds) and plant oils (flaxseed oil, soybean oil, canola oil). The optimal ratio of omega 6 to omega 3 in the diet is 3:1. Excessive amounts of omega 6 polyunsaturated fat and very high omega 6 to omega 3 ratio promotes the development of many diseases, including cardiovascular disease, cancer, and inflammatory and autoimmune diseases, whereas a lower omega 6 to omega 3 ratio reduces the risk of these disease conditions.[11]

The worst type of dietary fat is the trans fat. Unlike other dietary fats, trans fat lowers HDL cholesterol and raises LDL cholesterol levels. It is a by-product of a process called hydrogenation whereby oil is converted to a solid form by adding hydrogen. This process can occur in nature (natural trans fats) or in industries (artificial trans fat). Trans fats have no known health benefits. Natural trans fats occur in small amounts in meat and dairy products. Dietary sources of artificial trans fat include solid margarine and 'spreads'. Similarly, trans fats may be found in some cookies, pastries, cakes, doughnuts, ice cream, frozen pizza, snack foods and other commercial foods. Because of the health risks, trans fat has been banned in several high-income countries. There is no ban in the UK, but in 2012 most supermarkets and fast food chains signed a voluntary agreement not to use artificial trans fats.

Three portions of oil are required per day. A portion is equivalent to one table spoon of vegetable oil, or low-fat mayonnaise.

3. Beef, fish, eggs, beans, pulses and other proteins

Protein group foods (beef, fish, eggs, beans, pulses and other proteins) are an important source of protein, vitamins and minerals. I have replaced 'meat' with 'ox' to have 'O' in the FOODS acronym. Beans and pulses are inexpensive sources of fibre and protein, and are lower in fats than animal sources of protein. Nuts are included within the protein group; they are also an important source of unsaturated fats but be careful of the balance of omega 6 to omega 3 essential fatty acids that they contain.

It is recommended that you eat more beans and pulses because they are lower in fat and higher in fibre than animal proteins. Eat at least two portions of fish (2 × 140 g) per week, one of which should be oily fish. Oily fish, such as salmon, sardines, mackerel, whitebait and trout, are a source of omega-3 fatty acid.

Avoid processed meats and restrict intake of meat generally to not more than 70 g per day. Eating more than 70 g of red meat (beef, lamb, pork) and processed meat (sausages, bacon, ham, cured meats) per day has been associated with an increased the risk of bowel cancer. Meat is also high in saturated fats. 70 g of meat or poultry is equivalent to a piece of steak about the size of a deck of cards, three average-sized rashers of bacon or slices of ham, or a quarter-pounder beef burger.

About one third of the total daily food intake can come from the protein group and dairy/alternatives group The number of portions of the protein group depends on your daily calorie requirements (2500 kcal for men and 2000 kcal for women). A portion is equivalent to:
- 80 g of beans and pulses (3 heaped table spoons) or
- 140 g of fish or
- one egg (or 2 egg whites) or
- 25 g (1 tablespoon) of nuts or seeds or peanut butter.

4. Dairy and alternatives

Dairy and alternatives are important sources of protein, vitamins, calcium and iodine (but fish and seafood are a better source of iodine). This group includes milk, yoghurt, cheese, and calcium-fortified alternatives such as soya drink, soya yoghurt, nut milk, oat milk and rice milk. Some dairy products are high in saturated fats. Hence, go for the low-fat, low-sugar versions.

It is currently recommended that you eat three portions of low-fat dairy products or alternatives per day. A portion is equivalent to:
- a cup of milk or
- a cup of yoghurt or
- 42.5 g (1.5 oz) cheese.

Drink about 1.5 to 2 litres (6 to 8 glasses) of water per day. 'Water' includes water, low-fat milk and sugar-free drinks, including tea and coffee.

5. Starchy carbohydrates

One third of our total food intake can come from starchy carbohydrates, another one third from fruit and vegetables, and the last third from the dairy/alternatives and/or protein groups. Starchy foods are important sources of energy, fibre, B vitamins including folate (vitamin B9), iron, and calcium. It is important that you choose wholegrain, high-fibre varieties such as wholemeal bread, potatoes with skin and brown rice.

It is recommended that 50% of your daily calories come from starchy foods. The UK Eatwell guide recommends that we base our diet on starchy carbs, but to reverse diabetes, I found that consuming less carbohydrate and more protein and/or fat worked better. In order to reverse diabetes, I reduced my total calories by 50% and the remaining calories were mainly proteins and fats with just about 20% from carbs. I believe that excessive consumption of carbs may be the cause of the rapidly growing pandemic of type 2 diabetes. You should restrict your refined

sugar intake and aim to consume at least 30 grams of fibre per day. A portion in this group is equivalent to:
- 180 g of rice or
- 220 g of spaghetti or
- 60 g of potatoes or
- 2 slices of bread or
- 45 g of muesli.

The number of portions you have should depend on your daily calorie requirements (2500 calories for men and 2000 calories for women). Alcohol and sugary drinks contain a lot of calories and can therefore cause weight gain.

What to eat more of and what to avoid

There are three essential food types that most people do not eat enough of. I call them the 3Fs of Friendly foods: fruit and vegetables, fish and fibre. Make sure you have enough of the 3Fs in your diet. All natural, unprocessed starchy carbs, fruit and vegetables are rich in fibre.

On the other hand, there are foods that make people unwell and unfortunately people tend to overeat them. I call them the 3Ss of 'Sickness-causing' foods: salt, spreads and sugars. You should avoid the 3Ss as much as possible. The content of food 'spreads' varies widely and may include margarine, butter, mayonnaise, spreadable processed cheese, mustard, ketchup, nuts and seeds spreads and yeast extracts. Some have high levels of cholesterol and trans fat, and should therefore be avoided.

Note: The diet of a pregnant woman is similar to a balanced diet of non-pregnant woman. Do not increase calories during pregnancy. It's only in the last 12 weeks of pregnancy that you will need an extra of 200 calories per day. Do not try to lose weight during pregnancy. You will need iron and folic acid supplementation to prevent anaemia and birth defects.

3 Fs of 'friendly' foods

- Fruit and vegetables
- Fish (including oily fish)
- Fibre

3 Ss of 'sickness-causing' foods

- Salt
- Spreads
- Sugar

National food guides have failed to halt the obesity pandemic

National food guides provide guidance on how many portions (UK) or servings (US) of each food group should be consumed per day. These food guides also explain what is meant by a portion or serving. I recommend that you find your country's food guide on the internet. *The Eatwell Guide* is the UK food guide and *Myplate* is the US version. These guides are updated regularly and so you should keep up to date with the latest editions for your country. These guides are prepared by experts based on decades of scientific research, yet remain contraversial with regard to important issues, such as the dispute over sugar/carbs versus fat which has been going on for decades.

The UK *Eatwell Guide* recommends that you base your meals on starchy foods. As mentioned earlier in this chapter, significantly cutting down carbs is important to reverse type 2 diabetes (based on my experience) and I believe that it's also important to *prevent* type 2 diabetes. There is flexibility as to the balance between starchy carbs and proteins. This flexibility allows people to vary the amount of starchy carbs and proteins they take depending on their daily energy requirements.

The national food guides are developed by experts with the good intention of tackling some of the food-related health problems such as nutrient deficiencies and obesity. The intention may be good but the results are not.

Worldwide obesity has tripled in the last four decades. This shows that despite good intentions, national food guides have failed to achieve a major goal of preventing obesity. Overeating develops gradually. As children we are told to finish everything on our plate, and we gradually lose the ability to recognise when we are full. Many people eat far more calories than their body needs. Our stomach responds by expanding, getting bigger and bigger to contain the extra food. The body tries to overcome the effect of overeating by absorbing less food when you eat.[12] Our gut is like a washing machine in that it functions better when it is not completely full.

The rapid rise in type 2 diabetes and high blood pressure worldwide is evidence that the human body is rejecting the obesity culture

As we continue to overeat, this becomes a habit. Many have embraced this habit and it has become a widely accepted culture. Obesity is now a new normal. The rapid rise in type 2 diabetes and high blood pressure worldwide is evidence that the human body is rejecting the obesity culture. This is also evidence that national food guides are not achieving the intended results. Either people are eating less fat and more carbs, according to national food guides, and are getter fatter and fatter or they are not following the food guides – or perhaps a bit of both.

Chapter Four

Overweight and obesity

I was overweight and had both type 2 diabetes and high blood pressure. I had many friends who were obese, but were healthy with no diabetes or high blood pressure.

> **Lesson 4**
>
> Excess body fat (as seen in people who are overweight) can cause ill health even if you are not obese.

When I was diagnosed with hypertension and type 2 diabetes I had many friends who were either overweight or obese. As a physician, I realised most of my patients were also overweight or obese. Overweight and obesity were (and still are) so common that I had started questioning the scientific evidence behind the concept of what was a healthy weight. If almost everyone is fat, should being fat not be considered normal?

Despite my medical knowledge, my mind gradually accepted the fact that being fat was not a big problem. Indeed, I knew so many people who were fat and completely healthy that I concluded: 'It's the science that is wrong in this case. Science can't claim that almost everyone is too fat. How can everyone I see be overweight or obese? There must be something wrong with the definition of overweight and obesity.'

In my subconscious mind, I was fully convinced that being overweight – as opposed to obese – was not a problem. I recalled the difficulties I had had operating on obese women and that after the surgery their wounds took longer to heal. I therefore had little doubt that obesity was a cause of concern, but I reasoned: 'Overweight shouldn't be a problem. It's obesity that one should avoid.' Most 'normal' people I met were overweight. I thought that scientists should move the cut-off points upward for overweight and obesity so as to include more people currently considered overweight in the normal range.

When I was diagnosed with diabetes and high blood pressure, it didn't initially occur to me that the two conditions were caused by being overweight or having excess body fat because I knew so many people who were overweight or obese without health problems. Why should I develop ill health due to being overweight, while obese people had no health issues?

Overweight and obesity have been downplayed for too long and now we are heading towards a global catastrophe

When I lost 10 kg of my weight, my diabetes disappeared and I stopped taking medicine for it. The response of my diabetes to weight loss was a significant revelation. Excess body fat can cause type 2 diabetes even when you are not obese. From that moment, I understood why scientists had maintained the definitions of overweight and obesity for decades despite the fact that most people were now in those categories. Overweight and obesity are now indisputably a global pandemic. Some people argue that this pandemic has been exaggerated and I was one of them. After my personal experience, however, I switched to the other side of the argument. I am now fully convinced that the problems associated with being overweight or obese have been downplayed for too long and that we are heading towards a global catastrophe.

Chapter Four

It's not completely clear why some people tend to develop poor health due to overweight or obesity while others do not, but genetic factors, the location of fat stores in the body and the level of physical activity partly explain this apparent discrepancy. I was physically inactive and my fat location was abdominal (in the belly), both of which can increase the risk of sick fat disease.

I have also come to realise that there are widespread misconceptions about obesity. These myths are pervasive in the media, popular culture and even the scientific literature. Such myths include 'exercising is better than dieting to lose weight', 'obese individuals are less active than their normal-weight counterparts', 'calorie restriction works in the long term', 'eating more fruit and vegetables will make you lose weight', 'obesity is a sign of a good life', and many more. You will find hundreds of these misconceptions out there on the internet.

In order to lose weight, I decided to take control over my own health and weight loss. Rather than just being tele-guided by the many 'how-to' guides found on the internet, I decided to first understand more about what happened to the food I ate, how it was stored and burnt, how excess food caused overweight and obesity, and what could be done about it. I have summed up my experience into the following key points which are important for anyone who wants to lose weight or prevent themselves becoming overweight or obese:

- The body burns carbs and fats for fuel
- Overeating causes obesity
- Burning fats causes weight loss
- Excess abdominal fat causes sick fat disease
- Energy requirements reduce with age
- Processed foods make you overeat
- Exercise contributes to weight loss
- The ABCDE of weight loss provides a clear guide
- Orthorexia and other eating disorders must be borne in mind.

The body burns carbs and fats for fuel

Our body is like a car. It needs fuel to operate. Just like a hybrid car powered by diesel and a battery, our body gets its energy from carbohydrates and fats. If both fat and carbohydrate are available, our body prefers carbohydrate because it is easier and quicker to use. Once carbohydrate has been exhausted, the body turns to fat as the source of energy.

Our body burns starchy or long-chain carbohydrates in stages. The first stage is to break it down into the simple sugar called glucose. Then glucose in the blood triggers the pancreas to secrete the hormone insulin. In the second stage, insulin carries blood sugar into our cells where it is burnt to provide energy.

Any excess sugar is stored as glycogen in the liver and muscles. The glycogen store is relatively small and most people can only take up to a maximum of 600 grams of glycogen, although people with more muscle mass can store considerably more than that. When the glycogen store is full, excess sugar is converted and stored as fat. Body fat cells ('adipose tissue') and glycogen are therefore the two body stores for excess carbohydrates and fats. Adipose tissue is a bigger store that can take unlimited amounts of fat.

When glucose is depleted, the body turns to the liver and muscles for glycogen in the first instance. Glycogen is converted back to sugar by another hormone called glucagon, also produced by the pancreas. Glycogen can be seen as clusters of glucose molecules kept ready in the liver and muscles. Both insulin and glucagon are 'key workers' that regulate the amount of sugar in our blood, putting it into and out of storage.

If you continually overeat, your body will prioritise sugar and glycogen for energy and will almost never touch your body fat

If you continually eat carbohydrates in excess, your body will prioritise sugar and glycogen for energy and will almost never touch your body fat stores. Meanwhile, any excess sugar will be stored as glycogen and fat, and the cycle continues. Over time, the fat builds up in your body and you become overweight and then obese. Your body will only use fat for energy if there is no sugar or glycogen available. If you keep on eating more carbs than you need, and especially if you keep on snacking, there will never be an opportunity to take fat out of store.

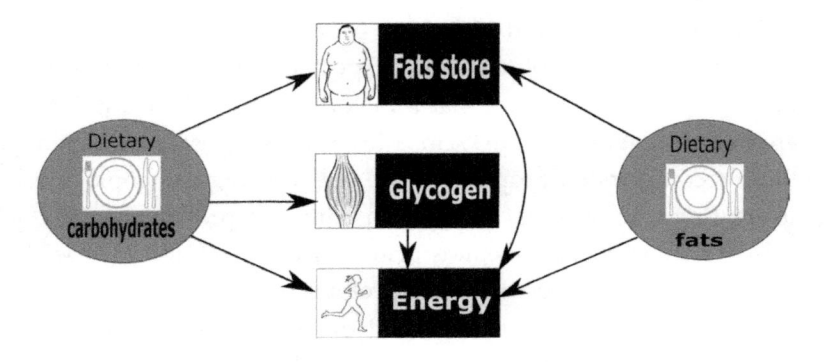

Figure 5: How the body burns and stores energy

A diet excessively high in pasta, bread, rice, soda, cornmeal, cassava, yam, wheat, millet, sorghum, barley, rye, and other carbs is a major risk factor for '*sick fat disease*' and fatty liver disease. We all know that *foie gras* ('fatty liver') is obtained by force-feeding geese with corn through a feeding tube to give them fatty livers. To obtain *foie gras*, corn is used, not fats. The same principle applies to humans. Excess carbs are transformed into fat.

Overeating causes obesity

Commonsense tells us that excessive consumption of either fats or carbs or both can cause obesity. Both fats and carbs when taken in excess are stored as fat in the body.

Obesity is caused by eating too much carbohydrate and too much fat – too much of almost everything

Obesity is more of a quantity problem rather than a quality problem. It is caused by eating too much carbohydrate and too much fat – too much of almost everything. Some experts recommend that 50% of total daily energy intake should come from carbs, 35% from fat and 15% from protein. Data from the UK show that most people tend to respect this recommendation fairly well. Given the fact that a majority of people in the UK are overweight or obese (63% in 2018),[13] this suggests that either these recommended proportions are not working or people are overeating both carbs, fat and protein. Although protein provides 15% of total energy intake, it is primarily used to build muscles and to make hormones and other proteins that the body needs.

It's self-evident that obesity and overweight are caused by people eating high-calorie foods, particularly carbohydrates and/or fats. So, in order to address the problem, we need to cut back on what we eat while making sure that we continue to consume enough fruit and vegetables and do not feel hungry.

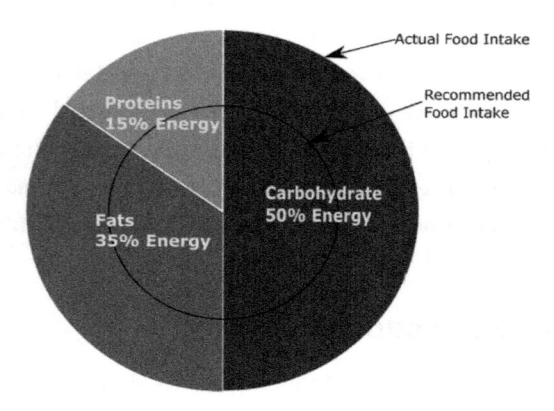

Figure 6: The difference between what we eat (outer ring) and what we need to eat (inner ring)

Chapter Four

Fat-burning causes weight loss

In order to burn fat and lose weight, we must significantly reduce both carbohydrate and fat intake. Once our glycogen store is depleted, the body is forced to burn fats for energy, as I have said. Burning fat for fuel instead of glycogen will lead to weight loss.

Fats are converted to ketones to provide fuel for the body. The process by which the body burns ketones for fuel is called *'ketosis'*.

Apart from weight loss, there are several other advantages of burning fat instead of glucose/glycogen for energy. The burning of body fat decreases appetite, reduces sugar cravings, increases HDL cholesterol, decreases LDL cholesterol, reduces blood sugar levels and reduces blood pressure.

One negative is that you may at first develop bad breath due to the burning of fats. This often disappears after some time, but if the problem persists, you can use any known brand of mouthwash or – my favourite – bicarbonate of soda (a tablespoonful in half a glass of water), to do away with the bad odour. Gargle it around your mouth for at least 30 seconds.

I lost 12.5% of my weight by reducing my carbs, fat and protein intake by 50%

To lose weight, I recommend that you significantly reduce your energy intake from carbs. In order to lose weight, I reduced my total calorie intake by 50% and I significantly reduced my carb intake compared to fat and protein. My calories from carbs reduced from about 50% to about 20% of my total calorie intake. As a result, I lost 12.5% (10 kg) of my weight – without feeling hungry!

Limiting food intake is difficult. From my experience, intermittent fasting is the easiest way to lose weight (see page 63).

First, when you fast, your stomach shrinks and so you will start eating less food than before. Second, fasting helps the body to switch from burning glycogen to burning fat. Third, when you have established a fasting routine, you will no longer be hungry while fasting.

Some people may find it difficult to fast for 14 to 16 hours. (This means eating dinner but skipping breakfast, for example.) Instead of fasting, you can try skipping your lunch as I did. Some will choose to skip breakfast instead. If you skip breakfast, make sure that your diet is not deficient in foods/nutrients normally eaten for breakfast. Overall, intermittent fasting is a good strategy to help you lose weight.

Make sure that you maintain a balanced diet as you downsize to a smaller plate. To ensure this, reduce mainly carbs and fats, and make sure you eat the recommended daily portions or servings of fruit and vegetables, oils and dairy or dairy-alternatives.

When fasting, make sure you drink enough water. Do not restrict your water intake. Water helps in the burning of fats, removes body waste, increases metabolism, suppresses your appetite, and helps during exercise. However, don't over-do it because excessive drinking of water flushes out essential minerals.

Excess abdominal fat causes sick fat disease

The body mass index, or BMI, is the measure of body fat based on the height and weight of a person. It is calculated as body weight (in kilograms) divided by the square of body height (in metres). It is expressed in units of kg/m^2.

- Underweight = BMI less than 18.5
- Normal weight = BMI 18.5 to 24.9
- Overweight = BMI 25 to 29.9
- Obese = BMI equal to or greater than 30

Chapter Four

Globally, over 50% of adults are overweight or obese by this reckoning. However, the BMI doesn't take into account the location of fat stores in the body though this is more important than the total amount of fat. While you have much control over the total amount of fat in your body, you have little control over where fat is stored. Your genes, gender, stress levels and age have more control over this.

Lower body or pear-shaped obesity

Upper body or apple-shaped obesity

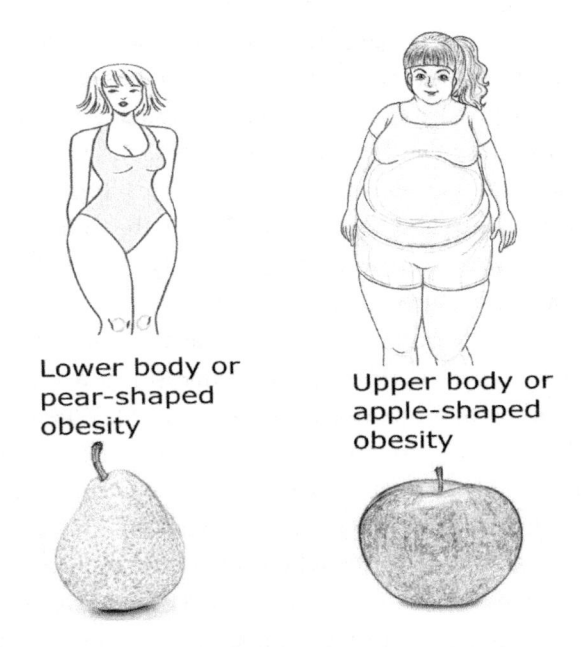

Figure 7: Pear-shaped versus apple-shaped obesity

As I have said, the two main locations for fat stores in the body are the upper body (abdomen) and the lower body (hips and thighs). The upper body or abdominal obesity is also called 'apple-shaped obesity' because the body shape is rounded like an apple. The lower body obesity is also called 'pear-shaped' obesity because the body shape looks like a pear (heavier lower down).

Apple-shaped obesity increases the risk of sick fat disease while pear-shaped obesity reduces this risk

Once the lower body store is full, fat will spill over to the abdominal organs leading to upper body obesity. Upper body obesity is also called abdominal or visceral or 'bad' or 'apple-shaped' obesity. Fat stores are located internally in the abdomen around the visceral organs and free fatty acids released from visceral fat can easily make their way into the liver where they can influence the production of blood lipids. Free fatty acids reaching the liver can be converted into LDL cholesterol. The LDL cholesterol increases the risk of diabetes, high blood pressure, heart disease and cancer. The liver is the body's chemical factory and if it fails to work properly, this affects all the other organs and makes the situation even worse.

Excessive consumption of fructose has been linked to non-alcoholic fatty liver. Table sugar (or sucrose) is a disaccharide (sugar that has two monosaccharide residues). When digested, it is broken down into fructose and glucose, yet only fructose has been strongly associated with the development of fatty liver disease. Whether fructose alone can cause this problem or if it serves only as a contributor when consumed excessively in the context of obesity and sedentary lifestyle is unknown. Due to excessive consumption of table sugar and sweetened foods, the global prevalence of non-alcoholic fatty liver disease in children and adolescents is escalating and currently represents the most common chronic liver disease in these groups.[14]

Body fat distribution explains why the BMI is not very accurate in predicting the risk of sick fat disease; it gives a reasonably accurate reflection of body fat, but doesn't tell the whole story. It doesn't tell us where the fat is located.

Some body hormones or 'key workers' influence the distribution of body fat. Low levels of sex hormones (testosterone and oestrogen) are associated with apple-shaped obesity. Similarly, high levels of cortisol, a hormone released by the adrenal glands, are associated with apple-shaped obesity. Cortisol levels tend to be chronically high during chronic stress and so stress can contribute to 'bad' obesity.

Hormone replacement therapy (HRT) is the use of oestrogen, or combined oestrogen and progestogen, to reduce the symptoms of menopause and bone loss after menopause. Some women decline to take HRT because they fear it causes weight gain. The current scientific evidence[14a] shows that HRT does not have any effect on body weight additional to that usually gained at the time of menopause. If you eat a low carb diet and maintain the same level of physical activity, it's unlikely that you will put on weight at menopause, although fat distribution may change in favour of the abdominal region.

Energy requirements reduce with age

Body energy requirements are influenced by aged. Our energy requirements increase from age 1 to 18 years, and then decrease progressively thereafter. Children and adolescents need energy for growth. Adults need energy for maintenance. Basal metabolic rate, or BMR, is the number of calories required to keep your body functioning at rest. Both the BMR and total energy requirement increase to the age of 18 years and then fall progressively with age.

During the last two decades, there has been a focus on the quality of our diet. However, the quantity dimension has not been effectively publicised yet it is this that seems to be driving the obesity pandemic (the number of calories we eat) rather than the quality. To prevent obesity, we must check the quantity to ensure that we do not overeat high-calorie foods, while keeping an eye on the quality (so that we have the required amount of vitamins and minerals).

For this reason, adults should in general eat less than teenagers. Unfortunately, this is often not the case for many reasons.

First, teenagers are dependent on adults for food and may not get enough, especially when they are in schools away from home. Once a teenager becomes an adult, he or she starts working and earning his or her own money. Adulthood is the time to eat less, but with more money it may be difficult to cut back on food intake.

Table 3: Average energy requirements by age

Age in years	Males (kcal)	Females (kcal)
1 year	765	717
5 years	1482	1362
10 years	2032	1936
15 years	2820	2390
18 years	3155	2462
19-20 years	2772	2175
25-34 years	2749	2175
35-44 years	2629	2103
45-54 years	2581	2103
55-64 years	2581	2079
65-74 years	2342	1912
75+ years	2294	1840

Second, adults tend to exercise less compared with children and teenagers, who tend to be relatively more active at home and in playgrounds. Physical activity increases energy consumption both during activity and while at rest after the activity.

Third, changing the eating habits established during teenage-hood is difficult. The consequence is that young adults continue to eat as if they were teenagers, or even more. In some cultures, the amount of food served to adults, especially men, is three times the amount given to teenagers. Overeating is likely to continue throughout the person's lifetime if no deliberate action is taken. The excess food is stored as fat. Overtime, this causes sick fat disease comprised, as we have seen, of obesity, high cholesterol, high blood pressure and eventually diabetes.

Processed foods make you overeat

The two most important hormones or 'key workers' involved in regulating hunger and satiety are *ghrelin* and *leptin*. Ghrelin, or the 'hunger hormone', is produced by the stomach when the body needs energy. It enters the 'feeding centre' of the brain (in the hypothalamus) and activates hunger.

In contrast to ghrelin, leptin – produced by fatty ('adipose') tissue – regulates satiety. Leptin, or the 'satiety hormone', reduces hunger by stimulating the 'satiety centre' of the brain (again in the hypothalamus).

Processed food, with added sugar, salt and fat, impairs the responses of leptin (the satiety hormone) and ghrelin (the hunger hormone) and causes people to overeat

Processed food, with added sugar, salt and/or fat, impairs leptin and ghrelin responses, Processed food has been shown to induce leptin resistance.[14] and causes people to overeat, partly by inducing such resistance.[15] Scientists have found that 'ultra-processed' foods led people to eat more and put on weight.[15] Therefore, in order to limit obesity, you should avoid processed food.

'Processed' carbohydrates go through a manufacturing process that removes fibre and breaks down the complexity of their natural chains. The elimination of complexity allows them to be easily digested and rapidly raises blood sugar. On the other hand, complex natural carbs, such as whole grains and cereals, take time to digest and provide vitamins, minerals and fibre

– both soluble (which we can ferment) and insoluble. Fibre maintains bowel health, lowers cholesterol levels and helps control blood sugar levels. Ultra-processed foods are highly processed and made mostly from substances extracted from whole foods, such as fats, plus added sugars, starches and hydrogenated fats.

Processed food is food that have been altered in some way during preparation, by heating (e.g. pasteurisation, homogenisation), freezing, sweetening, canning, baking, hydrogenation or drying. Not all processed foods are bad though. For example, pasteurising milk destroys harmful bacteria. What makes processing bad is the removal of fibre or the adding of sugar, salt and/or fat. For example, sugar is added to cakes, puddings and many savoury products and salt is added to bread. Whole-wheat bread is better because it is made of flour from whole-wheat grains that include fibre, although it may also have other added substances for preservation or colouring. On the other hand, white bread is made of flour from which fibre has been removed.

I couldn't agree more with Laurie Ellen David, an American environmental activist, when she said: *'Food is purposefully formulated to addict you. Then it is purposefully marketed, targeted to young children to addict them at an early age. This is unethical, right? This is immoral, particularly when you see the results of it which is a worldwide epidemic of diabetes and obesity.'*

Exercise contributes to weight loss

Obesity is a result of too many calories in, and too few calories burnt. Calories are is the unit for energy. Excess energy food is stored as fats, as I have said. Exercise is one of the most important factors that determine how much energy is burnt. Keeping active can help people maintain a healthy weight and lower the risk of sick fat disease.

Despite the health benefits of physical activity, people are less active today than they were even a few decades ago. This physical inactivity is due to changing lifestyles, with an increase in sedentary activities such as watching television, playing video-games and working on computers.

How much exercise do you need to prevent obesity? Most guidelines recommend 150 to 300 minutes per week of moderate intensity (or 75 to 150 minutes of vigorous intensity) to reduce the risk of heart disease, stroke, type 2 diabetes and cancer.

How much physical activity do you need to lose weight? Exercise can help you lose weight, but don't expect to lose much from exercise alone. While it has many health benefits, how much and what we eat has a much bigger impact on our weight. You burn an equivalent of two slices of pizza after one hour of moderate-intensity exercise. While 100% of our weight comes from food, only 10 to 30% can be burnt by exercise. Therefore, we must combine exercise, calorie reduction and a decrease in carbs if we want to reasonably lose weight.

First 20/80 rule:
Weight loss is achieved 80% by dieting and 20% by exercising

In my case, I estimate that 80% of my weight loss was due to calorie reduction and 20% to exercise. I call this my 'First 20/80 Rule'. Exercise, however, is important because of its numerous health benefits, including lowering high blood pressure.

In addition to exercise, you need to remain active throughout the day. (I talk more about the distinction between 'exercise' and 'physical activity' in Chapter 8.) You can use a standing work station to remain active while at work. At home, do some manual activities, such as cooking, cleaning, gardening etc, to remain active.

Note: During pregnancy, do not diet or try to lose weight but keep active; aim to do 150 minutes of exercise of moderate intensity every week.

The ABCDE of weight loss

Sticking to national food guides can help to prevent obesity. However, if you are already obese or overweight, you need to do much more than just follow the guides. It took me three months to lose 10 kg and I have sustained that weight loss for seven years now. I sum up my experience and the lessons I learnt about weight loss with what I call the **ABCDE** of weight loss:

- **A** = Abstain
- **B** = Balance
- **C** = Cut back
- **D** = Drink
- **E** = Exercise

1. Abstain

Intermittent fasting or abstaining from food is one of the easiest ways to reduce total food intake. By fasting for 14 to 16 hours a day, your body is depleted of glycogen. Glycogen-burning is switched to fat-burning, which leads to weight loss. Fasting has many advantages, including the fact that you get less hungry when fasting and your stomach shrinks so that you eat less food when you break the fast.

Eat two or three meals a day, but don't have any snacks between those meals. When fasting, all your meals should be eaten within a period of eight to 10 hours and nothing between those meals. Having snacks, whether they are healthy or not, increases your calorie intake and stimulates you to keep producing insulin, exacerbating insulin resistance.

2. Balance

To lose weight you need to cut back your food and/or calorie intake. As you downsize your plate, you must make sure that you maintain a balanced diet in terms of consuming all the essential nutrients you need. In order to ensure that your diet remains healthy, reduce mainly your carb and fat intake, and make sure you consume the recommended daily portions or servings of vegetables.

You may realise that you are/were disproportionately overeating carbohydrates. This means that you have to reduce these more than the other food groups. The same holds for fats. I found that basing my diet on proteins and/or fats was more effective in losing weight than basing it on carbs. I successfully lost 10 kg by reducing my total calories by 50% and the proportion of calories from carbs to about 20%.

3. Cut back

You must significantly cut back on your total calorie intake (carbohydrates, fats and proteins) especially carbs. This will cause depletion of sugar and glycogen, and force your body to start burning fats. Do it gradually while bearing in mind that this is a life goal. You must maintain the new food habit after achieving your weight loss goal. As I have said, I lost 12.5% of my weight by reducing 50% of my total calorie intake (carbs, fats and proteins). I significantly reduced carbs compared with fat and protein, which I reduced just a little. Calorie restriction in principle should lead to weight loss, but in practice it's difficult for many people including myself to sustain it. It didn't work for me. However, restricting calories through intermittent fasting worked well for me because I wasn't feeling hungry when fasting. On the contrary, hunger drove me crazy when I restricted calories without fasting.

4. Drink

Drink enough water to help you lose weight. Drinking water helps in the burning of fats, removes body waste, helps during exercise, and suppresses your appetite. Drink at least 1.5 to 2 litres of water per day. What counts as 'water' includes low-fat milk, and sugar-free drinks such as tea and coffee. It's important to note that water-fasting even for religious reasons, can be associated with significant health risks. You should also be aware that overconsumption of water can cause other health problems, including the depletion of minerals as minerals get flushed out by the kidneys in urine.

5. Exercise

Exercise regularly to burn fat and increase your basal metabolic rate. You need 150 to 300 minutes per week of moderate to vigorous intensity exercise and to remain active throughout the day. The more exercise you take, the bigger the weight loss. If you can do more exercise than recommended, it's even better. I recommend that you consider doing more exercise if you want to lose weight or have been previously overweight and have lost weight. Exercise will add to the effect of intermittent fasting and you will lose weight faster.

Orthorexia and other eating disorders

It's important that you are aware of some important eating disorders, including orthorexia, bulimia, anorexia nervosa and binge eating because they may not only influence your efforts to lose weight, but can be life-threatening. Please consult your doctor immediately if you feel you may have any of these disorders. Although the exact cause of eating disorders is unknown, they are all treatable conditions and the sooner addressed the more likely is recovery.

While you try to adopt a healthy-eating lifestyle, it's important not to overdo it. Be aware of orthorexia which is on the rise. The term 'orthorexia', or 'orthorexia nervosa', refers to an obsession with healthy eating. People with this condition want to achieve optimal nutrition and compulsively check ingredients lists and nutritional labels, unable to eat anything but for a narrow group of foods that are considered 'healthy'. They experience high levels of distress when 'healthy' foods aren't available. Orthorexia involves restriction of the amount and variety of foods eaten and this predisposes the person to malnutrition. Studies have shown that many people with this condition also have obsessive-compulsive disorder (OCD), a mental health problem characterised by excessive thinking (obsessions) that lead to repetitive behaviours (compulsions). The cause of orthorexia is unknown, although some experts believe it is actually a manifestation of OCD rather than a separate condition.

Anorexia nervosa is a more widely known, potentially lethal, eating disorder, characterised by extreme weight loss, food restriction, fear of gaining weight and a strong desire to be thin. Many people with this condition believe they are overweight, even though they are actually underweight. Studies suggest that serotonin (a hormone that stabilises mood, and promotes feelings of well-being and happiness) may play a part in anorexia nervosa. Reduced activity of serotonin receptors in the brain, with lower binding to serotonin, have been reported in anorexia patients. Alterations in serotonin have been linked to traits characteristic of anorexia, such as obsessiveness, anxiety and appetite dysregulation. There is evidence that biological, psychological, developmental and sociocultural factors contribute to anorexia, but the exact cause remains unknown.

Bulimia nervosa (or simply 'bulimia') is a serious, potentially life-threatening eating disorder characterised by a cycle of binge eating and followed by purging (self-induced vomiting or taking laxatives) in an attempt to get rid of the food consumed. There is evidence that biological (including genetic predisposition) and social factors contribute to bulimia, but, like anorexia, the exact cause remains unknown. The drive for thinness has been reported as the major cause of purging, as a way of controlling weight in order to achieve the 'ideal' body weight often portrayed by the media. The suicide rate among people with bulimia nervosa is 7.5 times higher than in the general population.[17]

Binge eating disorder is a severe, life-threatening, eating disorder characterised by recurrent episodes of eating large quantities of food at once until the person feels uncomfortably full, and then often upset, depressed, guilty, ashamed and/or disgusted. People with bulimia nervosa and binge eating disorder exhibit similar patterns of compulsive overeating and food addiction, but bulimia is distinguished from binge eating by its characteristic purging. Binge eating is one of the most prevalent eating disorders among adults. The cause is not fully understood, although studies have suggested biological factors (including genes), traumatic life events, rigid eating practices or an expression of a deeper psychological problem, such as depression.

Chapter Five

Intermittent fasting

In order to lose weight, I stopped having lunch and snacks. I didn't respect any other rules about intermittent fasting. I lost 10 kilos in three months, and was stronger and healthier.

> **Lesson 5**
>
> Intermittent fasting is one of the easiest ways to lose weight, but its benefits go far beyond weight loss.

In order to lose weight, I first reduced my food/calorie intake without intermittent fasting. I lost only 1 kg, but hunger drove me crazy. I felt as though I was starving every day. After struggling with calorie reduction for several weeks, I concluded that it was not for me. The level of hunger I had experienced was unbearable. I finally gave up. This attempt failed because I couldn't reduce the quantity of calories I consumed enough, and I couldn't sustain the reduction. I got so hungry that I had to eat.

The second thing I tried was exercise. I tried 30 minutes, 60 minutes, 90 minutes and 120 minutes of walking every day, but didn't see any change in my weight. I tried jogging and running, and again found no significant change in my weight. I came to the conclusion that exercising was necessary but not sufficient to make me lose weight. Of course, the effect of exercise depends on its duration and intensity.

Finally, I decided to stop having lunch and snacks. It was a very big decision because lunch was my principal meal. I enjoyed it and used it to socialise with friends. I was used to taking it with my co-workers – it was more than just lunch. It was fun! Lunch was a time to relax and distract from the busy work schedule. Now, I still socialize with colleagues during lunch. My friends know and accept the fact that I don't eat lunch. I drink tea while they eat.

In addition to lunch, I also stopped having snacks. No more chocolates! When any of us travelled, we came back with chocolates for everyone. It was our work culture. My decision to stop lunch and snacks meant I would miss all the fun and merrymaking. However. my drive to find a solution to weight loss was far stronger than my feelings about what I was going to miss. And so I went ahead.

The first three days were the most difficult; this was when I stopped having lunch. At lunchtime I got very hungry and weak. To reduce the hunger, I drank more water to keep my stomach full, and had more tea and coffee without milk or sugar. After the first three days, the hunger reduced and, by the second week, my body had adapted to the new eating schedule.

I continued without lunch and snacks for the next three months. On weekends, it was much more difficult not to have lunch while staying at home. But with strong willpower, every Saturday and Sunday I avoided lunch and snacks. In three months, I had lost 10 kg, as I have said. I also noticed I ate less at dinner; my stomach shrank and I got full more quickly than before.

After three months, I read an article about intermittent fasting. It was then that I realised that by stopping having lunch I had been doing intermittent fasting off my own bat. When I had introduced my 'no lunch, no snacks' strategy, I hadn't known it was intermittent fasting.

Despite the fact that I didn't meet the minimum 14 hours of fasting every day, I got the same results as intermittent fasting. 'No lunch, no snacks' is therefore another way to fast and lose weight.

I then did an internet search for 'intermittent fasting' and got 55,300,000 hits. The internet is flooded with facts and misconceptions about intermittent fasting. Before you jump into such a plan, you need to distinguish fact from myth. I summarise the important things you need to know about this approach into five key points:

1. Fasting is an ancient tradition
2. Counting calories doesn't work
3. Intermittent fasting does work
4. Intermittent fasting has many health benefits
5. Try these intermittent fasting plans.

Fasting is an ancient tradition

Fasting is an ancient tradition that has been practised by many cultures and religions for a number of reasons, including for religious purposes, as a form of protest and for medical benefits.

1. Fasting for religious purposes

Fasting has been practised as part of religious observance since ancient times. It was, and is still, believed to bring people closer to God, reveal divine teachings through dreams and visions, cleanse people of their sins, assuage an angered deity, have the power to heal and bring blessings to the devotees.

Today, fasting is practised by many religions, including Christianity, Islam, Hinduism, Judaism and Buddhism. To Muslims, the month of Ramadan is a period of penitence and total fasting from dawn to dusk. Fasting is used in Judaism during the days of penitence or mourning. Catholic, some Anglican and Eastern Orthodox Christians observe fasting for penitence during Lent.

2. Fasting as a form of protest

Fasting has been used as a form of protest or solidarity, sometimes called a 'hunger strike'. It has been used to protest against wars, social evils and social injustice. Classic examples include the Suffragettes in the UK and US, seeking 'votes for women' Mahatma Gandhi's fast in prison in the early 20th century to make a point to his followers who didn't practise his teachings of non-violence against British rule in India. In the 1960s, Dick Gregory, an American Black comedian, fasted against the violations of civil rights of American Indians. In 1981, 10 Irish prisoners died in prison following a hunger strike to demand recognition of their status as political prisoners.

3. Medical fasting

Therapeutic fasting has been used at least since the time of the Greek physician, Hippocrates, considered the father of modern medicine. Hippocrates recommended fasting to patients who exhibited certain symptoms, including all fevers.

There was renewed medical interest in fasting in the 1960s for the treatment of obesity. Research tested different fasting periods ranging from 14 hours to 21 days.[18] Prolonged fasting was found to have some unpleasant side-effects in a few people, such as a significant fall in blood pressure when the person stood up (orthostatic hypotension). These side-effects prompted doctors to caution against prolonged fasting without adequate medical monitoring.

Chapter Five

There is a growing body of scientific knowledge that supports the use of intermittent fasting for weight loss and the treatment of diabetes.[19] Available scientific evidence shows that this type of fasting has a broad range of health benefits for many conditions, including obesity, diabetes, high blood pressure, heart disease, cancers and neurological disorders.

Why counting calories doesn't work

Many people have been told by 'experts' that, in order to lose weight, they need to calculate their calorie intake and calories burnt. They then spend time noting down everything they eat and the corresponding calories. They also estimate how many calories they have burnt throughout the day. Nowadays with smart phone apps it is far easier to do this. There are many apps that count your steps and will tell you how many you have taken, how far you have moved and how many calories you have used up at the end of the day.

The logic behind the 'calorie in, calorie out' concept is based on the fact that if you can take in fewer calories than you actually burnt, then you will lose weight.

Calorie intake = Calories burnt (Exercise) + Calories burnt (BMR)

The energy a person burns at rest is called their basal metabolic rate, or BMR. The thinking is that if you can know how many calories you take in, and how many you burn thanks to exercise and BMR, you can determine whether you are going to lose or gain weight. 'Excess calorie intake' means weight gain and 'excess calorie burning' means weight loss.

While this concept is simple in theory, in practice it is difficult to apply for many reasons:
1. First, many people struggle to calculate their calorie intake exactly. They may forget to note everything they

eat. They may not be able to find the exact calorie count for everything they do eat. They may need to weigh everything they eat which makes life difficult, or they may not have weighing scales to do this. And the list of problems encountered when trying to measure calorie intake continues (see Figure 8).

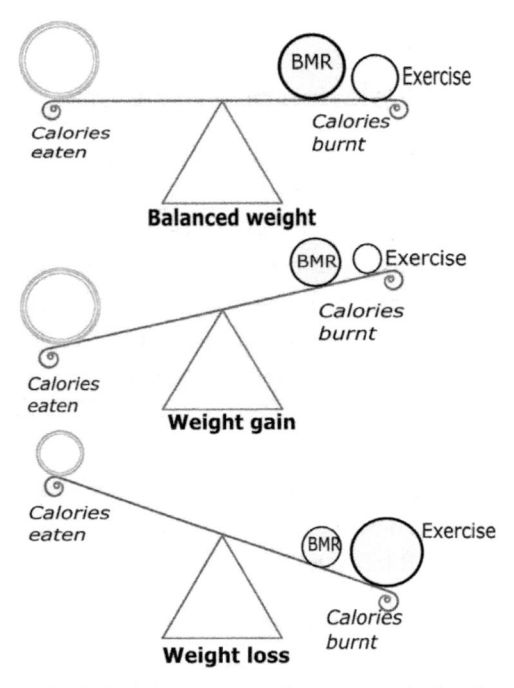

Figure 8: Calories consumed versus calories burnt

2. Second, one's basal metabolic rate is not fixed. The rate at which a person burns calories at rest (BMR) depends on the amount of calories consumed; the higher the calorie intake, the more calories are burnt at rest. For example, when a person decreases their calorie intake by 10%, their BMR decreases by 15%. Calorie intake and calorie burning are not independent of each other; they are

co-dependent. This means that if you reduce your calorie intake, you will not lose weight by an amount equal to the reduction in calories.

The more calories you eat, the more calories you burn at rest

3. Third, when I tried calorie reduction without intermittent fasting, it left me hungry throughout the day. That pushed me to snack in-between meals to control the hunger. As a result, I was unable to reduce the calories I consumed sufficiently to lead to any significant weight loss.[20]

This explains why many people struggle to lose weight. They reduce their food intake and yet they find that they do not lose weight. After several attempts at struggling with daily hunger due to food intake reduction, they finally give up.

'Counting calories' is a myth because we ignore the fact that when we reduce our food or energy intake, there is compensatory reduction in our basal metabolic rate and therefore a reduction in overall energy burnt.

Why intermittent fasting works

Intermittent fasting causes a metabolic switch from sugar burning to fat burning. When you are fasting, your body will first burn the available sugar in your blood for energy. Glycogen in your liver and muscles will be converted to sugar and burnt for energy also. Once the glycogen store is depleted, your body will turn to burning fat. The burning of fats leads to weight loss. How long it takes for your body to switch from glycogen to fat burning depends on how much glycogen you have in your liver and muscles.

After 10 to 12 hours of abstinence, most people have depleted their glycogen stores. Therefore, optimal results are obtained when you fast for more than 12 hours. Fasting for 14 to 16 hours is a generally accepted period for abstinence. Although fasting for longer than 16 hours may give results, it may cause orthostatic hypotension in some people and it is difficult to sustain in the long run. (As mentioned earlier, orthostatic hypotension is the fall in blood pressure below the normal range when a person stands up.)

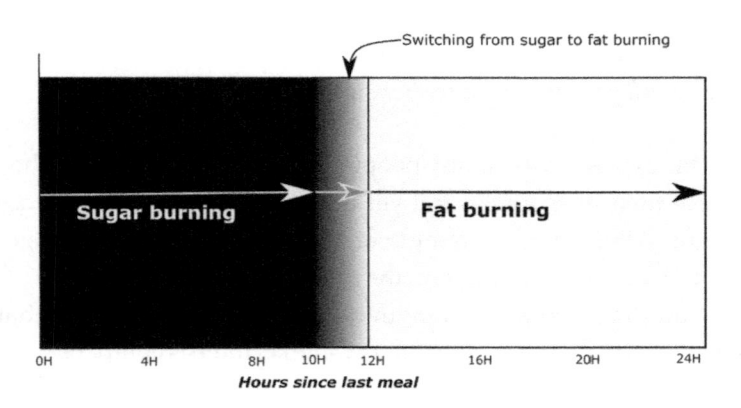

Figure 9: From sugar burning to fat burning

The first few days of fasting can be difficult because we are changing our natural clock which runs in the background at all times. This 24-hour internal clock is called our *'circadian rhythm'* and is controlled by part of the brain (the hypothalamus). After many years of behaving in a certain way, the body is used to its usual eating times and sleeping times. This becomes a cycle running in the background in our brain. Most people will take two to five days to completely break this cycle and adjust their clock to new eating times. Once the cycle has been broken we can establish a new routine which fits with our 24-hour internal

Chapter Five

clock. Changing the circadian rhythm by intermittent fasting brings about positive metabolic changes in our cells.

One of the positive changes due to the change in circadian rhythm is a reduction in blood levels of the hunger hormone, ghrelin, when fasting. During fasting, the levels of ghrelin are low. Ghrelin is secreted by the stomach when the body needs energy. Blood levels of ghrelin are highest just before meals and lowest just after them. Ghrelin seems to be released in waves. This means that a person who eats three times a day may have three waves of ghrelin increase in their blood. These waves of ghrelin correspond to the times the person normally eats. A person who is on intermittent fasting and eating twice a day will have only two peaks of ghrelin. Following each wave, ghrelin levels will decrease after approximately two hours without food consumption. Each ghrelin peak causes a wave of hunger which will recede as the ghrelin level drops, even if you don't eat. This explains why during fasting people do not feel continuously hungry.[21]

If we just reduce the amount of food we eat per meal without fasting, we spend most of the day hungry because our blood ghrelin levels are high. This is why many people can't sustain weight loss because they feel as though they are starving all day long. In practice, therefore, many people find it easier to reduce food intake by fasting because they are not hungry when fasting.

Intermittent fasting also causes the stomach to shrink in size. The stomach usually distends when we overeat eat to create space for the extra food consumed. The opposite occurs when we fast. Since the stomach stays for a long time without food, it reduces in size. When we break the fast, we eat less than we normally would because our stomach has shrunk.

However, please not that this is not a good idea when you are pregnant so do not do intermittent fasting if you are expecting a baby. Trying to lose weight when pregnant is not recommended.

Intermittent fasting has many health benefits

The metabolic switch from sugar to fat burning triggers a chain of events within the body that brings several health benefits. Intermittent fasting confers health benefits beyond weight loss. It reduces obesity, high cholesterol, high blood pressure, blood clot formation and inflammation and improves our sensitivity to insulin. It prevents heart disease, cancers and brain diseases. Just restricting calorie intake without fasting doesn't confer the same health benefits.

The following are some of the numerous health benefits of fasting:
- Ageing (slows)
- Blood pressure (normalises)
- Stress (becomes easier to cope with)
- Clot formation (normalises)
- Obesity (reduces)
- Neoplasm (cancer) (reduces risk)
- Diabetes, type 2 (reverses)
- Inflammation (asthma, arthritis, multiple sclerosis) (reduces)
- Neurodegenerative disorders (Alzheimer's, Parkinson's) (reduces risk)
- HDL cholesterol (increases).

1. Ageing

Intermittent fasting decreases the production of poisons called 'oxygen free radicals' by the body as part of our ongoing metabolic processes. The free radicals injure our cells and tissues by a process called *'oxidative stress'* which can alter our genetic code (also called 'gene mutation'), cause the death of body tissues (also called 'degeneration'), and lead to chronic inflammation, all of which lead to ageing. Intermittent fasting therefore slows ageing. Furthermore, it promotes the production of 'antioxidants', which are antidotes to the free radicals. The antioxidants neutralise the harmful free radicals and promote healthy growth of brain tissue. This improves memory and learning ability.

2. Blood pressure

Intermittent fasting lowers blood pressure by triggering a chain of events that flushes out sodium and causes vasodilation (widening of the arteries), both of which lower blood pressure.

3. Stress

The body responds to fasting by producing 'antioxidants' which are antidotes that neutralise free radicals, as just described, repair damaged genes, reduce inflammation and promote autophagy. 'Autophagy' is the process by which our cells remove or recycle unnecessary or dysfunctional parts – a form of 'spring cleaning'. The functioning of the body during fasting is significantly improved. The fasting cells develop strong resistance to potentially damaging attacks and all forms of internal disorder.

4. Clot formation

High levels of free fatty acids and cytokines (the body's police), as a result of being overweight or obese, as we have seen, increases the formation of blood clots (thrombosis). Intermittent fasting reduces free fatty acids, cytokines and inflammation and thereby prevents abnormal blood clot formation. This reduces the risk of life-threatening conditions caused by blood clots that block the blood supply to the heart (heart attack), brain (stroke) and lungs (pulmonary embolism).

5. *Obesity*

The switch from burning sugar to fat directly leads to weight loss. One of the things that happens as a result of this switch is a change in our 24-hour internal clock or circadian cycle to adapt to the new eating routine. The fasting circadian cycle significantly lowers insulin levels, improves insulin sensitivity, lowers blood pressure and significantly decreased appetite. We feel less hungry when fasting and can consequently lose weight and actually maintain fasting as a new normal without feeling that we are starving.[22]

6. *Neoplasm (cancer)*

Preclinical studies have found that intermittent fasting reduces the risk of cancer.[23] In addition, fasting impairs energy metabolism in cancer cells, suppresses the growth of cancer cells and renders them more susceptible to clinical treatments, partly because they rely heavily on glucose rather than fat for energy.

Intermittent fasting has also been found to extend survival among cancer patients.[24]

7. *Diabetes*

Intermittent fasting reverses insulin resistance and thereby reduces the risk of type 2 diabetes. It also reverses type 2 diabetes. People who lose weight by calorie restriction do not experience the same level of improvement in type 2 diabetes that people undertaking intermittent fasting do because intermittent fasting promotes multi-system regeneration, including the regeneration of the pancreas.[25] This confirms that the benefits of intermittent fasting go far beyond those related to weight loss.

8. *Inflammation (asthma, multiple sclerosis, arthritis)*

Intermittent fasting reduces the symptoms of asthma in obese patients by reducing inflammation.[26]

Multiple sclerosis is an autoimmune disease in which the immune (defence) system through inflammation eats away the protective covering of the nerves resulting in nerve damage. Intermittent fasting reduces inflammation, improves immune (defence) function and prevents or delays the progression of multiple sclerosis.[26]

Rheumatoid arthritis is another autoimmune disease that is associated with inflammation, pain and damage to joints and can extend to other organs of the body. Intermittent fasting is also beneficial to patients with rheumatoid arthritis and other forms of arthritis because it reduces inflammation.

9. Neurodegenerative disorders

Excessive calorie intake increases the risks of Parkinson's disease and Alzheimer's disease, which are both neurodegenerative disorders, so-called because they are caused by the death of brain cells or tissue. Intermittent fasting delays the onset of both Parkinson's and Alzheimer's diseases.[26] It increases brain tissue resistance through gene repair, a decrease in inflammation, and autophagy (removal of unnecessary or dysfunctional parts of the cell).

10. HDL cholesterol

Intermittent fasting lowers low-density lipoprotein (LDL) cholesterol and increases high-density lipoprotein (HDL) cholesterol. LDL cholesterol can build up in blood vessels where there is an injury/damage due to oxidative stress and block blood flow. The blockage of blood flow to the heart causes heart disease. Fasting therefore reduces the risk of heart disease.

It's important to note that both HDL and LDL are heterogeneous and can be divided into sub-types based on their density and particle size. There are two types of LDL cholesterol according to the size of the LDL particles: type A (large dense LDL) and type B (small dense LDL). Type A LDL is considered to be dangerous and mostly likely to be associated with heart disease. Type B LDL can enter the arterial blood vessel walls where it becomes oxidised, causing inflammation. There are two types of HDL: HDL2 (larger, less dense) and HDL3 (smaller, denser). Both HDL2 and HDL3 have been found to predict lower risk for heart disease.[27]

Caution with fasting

While fasting has many benefits, it is not good for everyone. The following groups of people should not fast:
- Small and/or underweight (body mass index less than 18.5)
- Children
- Anyone with anorexia or another eating disorder
- Lactating and pregnant women
- Elderly and/or frail
- Those with diabetes type 1.

Intermittent fasting plans

There are several intermittent fasting plans. I regularly use the 'no lunch' version. I have tried out the '16-hour plan' and the '14-hour plan', both of which worked well, but my favourite is 'no lunch'. I haven't tried out the '24-hour plan', but some people prefer it. You can choose any of the four plans depending on your preference. Pick a plan that you will be able to stick to for the long term. If you stop intermittent fasting, you run the risk of regaining the weight you lost while fasting.

In all four plans, make sure that you don't have any snacks between meals. Having snacks raises blood insulin levels, which leads to insulin resistance and offsets the benefits of fasting.

Chapter Five

Drink a lot of water while fasting – do not water-fast. Drinking water helps with fat burning, removes body waste and suppresses your appetite. It is advisable to drink about 1.5 to 2 litres of water per day. However, be aware that excessive drinking of water can cause depletion of minerals.

The four intermittent fasting plans are: 16-hour intermittent fasting plan; 14-hour intermittent fasting plan; 24-hour intermittent fasting plan; no-lunch intermittent fasting plan.

1. 16-hour intermittent fasting plan

With this plan, you fast for 16 hours and eat all your meals within eight hours. The easiest way to do this would be to have a late breakfast so that you can extend the period from your last meal to your breakfast to 16 hours. For example:
- If you start eating at 7 am, stop eating at 3 pm. (eight-hour window),
- If you start eating at 9 am, stop eating at 5 pm. (eight-hour window), and
- If you start eating at 12 noon, stop eating at 8 pm. (eight-hour window).

2. 14-hour intermittent fasting plan

With a 14-hour intermittent fasting plan, you fast for 14 hours and eat all your meals within 10 hours. For example:
- If you start eating at 7 am, stop eating at 5 pm (10-hour window)
- If you start eating at 9 am, stop eating at 7 pm (10-hour window)
- If you start eating at 12 noon, stop eating at 10 pm (10-hour window).

3. 24-hour intermittent fasting plan

With 24-hour intermittent fasting, you choose two days in a week (say Monday and Thursday) on which you fast for 24 hours. The rest of the five days of the week you eat normally. For example, if you eat dinner at 7 pm today, you will fast until 7 pm the next day. For this plan to work, it is very important that you do not compensate for the fasting days by eating more during the non-fasting days. You want to reduce your total calorie intake by taking advantage of the 24-hour zero calorie intake during fasting. This plan will not allow your circadian rhythm to adjust unlike the 14-hour and 16-hour plans. However, the 24-hour plan can still contribute to the regeneration of the pancreas.

A variant of this plan is to restrict your calorie intake to 500 to 600 calories per day during the two days of fasting and eat normally during the other days of the week.

4. No-lunch intermittent fasting plan

The simple approach I followed was to skip lunch. With this approach, you forget about counting the number of hours of fasting. You simply have your breakfast and dinner normally, and skip having any lunch. You have your breakfast when you normally would and your dinner when you prefer, but avoid having lunch or snacks between the two meals. I tried out this plan without knowing I was doing intermittent fasting and it worked so well. I still use it today.

Chapter Six

Type 2 diabetes

After trying different pill-free treatment plans for type 2 diabetes, the only thing that finally worked for me was weight loss.

> **Lesson 6**
>
> Type 2 diabetes is a dietary disease; the cornerstone of its prevention or reversal is weight loss.

When my doctor told me I had type 2 diabetes I was shocked. The news was devastating because I knew the implications of the diagnosis. I knew that if not properly managed, it would almost inevitably lead to life-threatening complications.

After a period of reflection, I was prepared to face the condition, not passively, but actively by taking control. I was prepared to try out every possible intervention to uncover anything that could reverse it. As I explained in the Introduction, I tried out 30 things over a two-year period. The 30th thing I tried was to stop having lunch and snacks. By stopping doing that, I lost 10 kg in three months and the diabetes disappeared.

It was a thrilling discovery because I was able to stop taking metformin, my anti-diabetic medication. Other things such as exercise also helped, but it was clear that weight loss was the centerpiece of the reversal. To me this has far-reaching implications for the way physicians should counsel newly diagnosed diabetic patients. If someone had told me that I could stop taking anti-diabetic medicine by losing 10 kg, it wouldn't have taken me two years to reverse my diabetes.

My experience is not an isolated case. A group of UK scientists have found that most type 2 diabetic patients reversed their diabetes by losing 10 to 15 kg.[28] Losing weight should be the main focus for diabetes reversal. It's important to let people know clearly that weight loss works. This can be the driving force behind lifestyle change.

There are a lot of facts, myths and misleading claims about diabetes. I did an internet search for this condition and got 636 million hits. For an average person, the biggest challenge is how to separate wheat from chaff – what is good quality information and what is 'fake news'? Based on my experience as a physician and as a patient, I identified six important points about diabetes which I believe everyone should know.

- Consumption of excess carbs and calories causes type 2 diabetes
- Weight loss is the cornerstone of diabetes reversal
- Intermittent fasting helps you lose weight
- Exercise complements intermittent fasting
- Dietary fibre lowers blood sugar
- Alcohol, smoking and stress reduction also help.

Consumption of excess carbs and calories causes type 2 diabetes

Diabetes is a disease in which the blood sugar level becomes too high. There are two types of diabetes – type 1 and type 2. Type 1 is caused by lack of insulin, a hormone that keeps blood sugar low by helping the cells to take in sugar to be used for energy.

Chapter Six

Type 2 diabetes is caused by insulin resistance, a situation where the cells become increasingly insensitive to insulin. Among all cases of diabetes globally, 95% are type 2 and only 5% are type 1.

> *Hormones are our bodies' 'key workers', ensuring that essential work is done to keep us alive. The hormone insulin is the 'key worker' that delivers sugar into our cells*

Insulin is a hormone produced by the pancreas. Hormones (chemical messengers) are our bodies' 'key workers', ensuring that essential work is done to keep us alive. Insulin is the key 'worker' that delivers sugar into our cells.

I recall during the first wave of the coronavirus pandemic, the UK Government ordered people to stay at home and identified the key workers who were allowed to go to work because their services were considered essential for survival. Some of these essential workers were those delivering food and medicines to the vulnerable people who were ordered to stay at home. People with certain conditions, such as high blood pressure, diabetes and heart disease, and the elderly were not allowed to leave home even to buy the basic necessities. The key workers did the job for them by delivering food and medicines to them at home. Insulin does exactly the same thing for the body's cells. It delivers sugar (fuel) and has the key that opens the door for sugar to enter our cells.

How does insulin resistance develop? It is a complex process because insulin acts at multiple stages in carbohydrate metabolism. It facilitates the uptake of sugar into adipose (fat) and muscle cells by binding to insulin receptors found on the cell membranes. It also increases glycogen synthesis and decreases glycogen breakdown. It stimulates glucose breakdown (glycolysis) and inhibits glucose synthesis (gluconeogenesis) by the liver. It enhances the oxidative pathway whereby pyruvate (produced

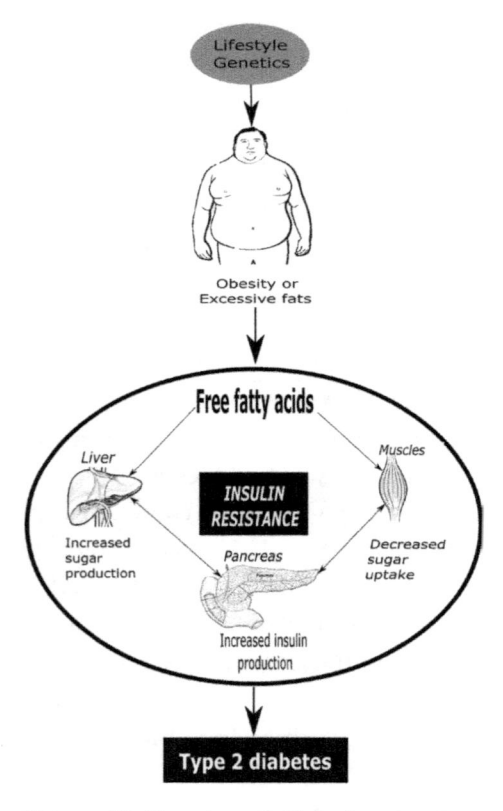

Figure 10: How type 2 diabetes develops

by glycolysis) is converted into acetyl Co-A in the mitochondria of the cells as part of energy production. Acetyl Co-A may then be either oxidised (via the downstream tricarboxylic acid cycle, known as Krebs' cycle) to produce energy or used for fatty acid synthesis.[29]

Chronic excess energy consumption promotes increased blood levels of insulin and insulin resistance through several factors, including:
- direct deleterious effects of excess carbs and excess fats on organs and tissues

- obesity-induced chronic inflammation
- activation of endoplasmic reticulum (ER) stress pathways.[30] (In cells, the structure called the endoplasmic reticulum serves multiple functions including the synthesis, folding, modification and transport of proteins.)

Excess calories have different effects on different tissues. Excess glucose and fats in the liver favour the shift from oxidative pathways that produce energy to esterification pathways that produce fats; these can activate enzymes (ser kinases) that inactivate insulin receptors by a process called phosphorylation. This inactivation ensures that the binding of insulin to its receptors does not generate any of the downstream effects described above (cellular glucose uptake, glycolysis, gluconeogenesis, etc). This too leads to insulin resistance.[30]

In muscle, excess lipids enhance fatty acid breakdown (oxidation) but do not induce Krebs' cycle (energy production). This leads to the accumulation of incompletely metabolised lipids (fats) in the cell mitochondria that can impair insulin signalling and further lead to insulin resistance.[30]

Obesity-induced chronic inflammation too causes insulin resistance. Excess calorie intake (whether from carbs or fat) can lead to overweight and obesity, as we have seen. Obesity can cause oxidative stress, a process by which excess oxygen free radicals injure body tissues and cells. How this happens is still incompletely understood, but one explanation is that obesity leads to the production of larger fatty cells (adipocyte hypertrophy and hyperplasia) which outstrip the local oxygen supply. This causes hypoxia (tissues starved of oxygen) and oxidative stress. Oxidative stress causes cell inflammation and the release of inflammatory cytokines, which also cause insulin resistance. (For those interested in the details, some examples of inflammatory cytokines include interleukin-1 (IL-1), IL-12, IL-18, tumour necrosis factor alpha (TNF-α), and interferon gamma (IFNγ).) Chronic inflammation in tissues can cause insulin resistance through the effect of cytokines on cells. Cytokines can act on the cells that produced them (autocrine signalling), diffuse and act on neighbouring cells (paracrine cytokine signalling) or enter blood circulation and affect cells in distant parts of the body (endocrine cytokine signalling).[30]

Excess uptake of carbs and fats causes an increase in insulin secretion, which ultimately leads to endoplasmic reticulum (ER) stress in pancreatic β-cells that results in loss of β-cell mass. Pancreatic β-cell are cells that produce insulin. As explained above, in the cell, the endoplasmic reticulum serves multiple functions including the synthesis, folding, modification and transport of proteins. Under these conditions of pancreatic β-cell loss, amylin, another product of the pancreas, is then secreted in excess so that it accumulates as amyloid plaques, causes β-cell damage and death. This leads to β-cell failure, signalling the onset of full-blown type 2 diabetes.[30]

In summary, there are multiple pathways that can lead to insulin resistance. All these are closely linked to excess calorie intake (carbs and fat). Ultimately, the final common pathway leading to insulin resistance may be the accumulation of fat and its intermediate products of metabolism in the liver and muscles. However, it's important to note that the main source of fat in the final common pathway of insulin resistance is excess dietary carbs/sugar and calories.[31]

Weight loss is the cornerstone of diabetes reversal

Type 2 diabetes is caused by insulin resistance (or insulin insensitivity). The high blood sugar level is a consequence or symptom of insulin resistance. Therefore, the ideal treatment for type 2 diabetes should be to treat the insulin resistance.

Antidiabetic medications such as metformin increase insulin sensitivity and therefore uptake and utilisation of sugar by the cells. In addition, metformin decreases the absorption of sugar by the intestines and the production of sugar by the liver. The liver can produce sugar either by breaking down glycogen or from byproducts of proteins and fat.

Injecting insulin is not the right treatment for type 2 diabetes. This is because patients with type 2 diabetes already have high levels of insulin in their blood. Giving insulin for type 2 diabetes can be likened to injecting drugs to relieve an addicted drug user from withdrawal symptoms. Drug users who are addicted to their drugs will start to have withdrawal symptoms if they don't take the drug after several hours. Withdrawal symptoms may include sweating, fatigue, anxiety, vomiting, depression, seizures and hallucinations. When experiencing withdrawal symptoms, the drug user will take the drug and experience immediate relief. Giving insulin to type 2 diabetics is similar. While increasing body insulin may provide some immediate benefits by forcing the uptake of sugar by the cells, this is counter-productive in the longer term. It can even make things worse by increasing insulin resistance. Yet, about one in four people with type 2 diabetes is put on insulin.

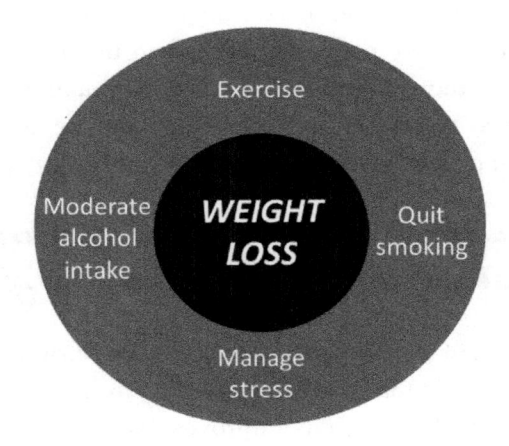

Figure 11: Weight loss is the cornerstone of type 2 diabetes reversal

The ideal treatment for insulin resistance is weight loss. Type 2 diabetes is a dietary disease and should therefore be treated through diet. Weight loss means fat loss. Weight loss improves insulin sensitivity and lowers blood sugar, thereby lowering blood insulin levels. Our cells can get the energy they need and our organs can start functioning normally.

Intermittent fasting helps you lose weight

Weight loss is central to the treatment of type 2 diabetes. Any dietary plan that doesn't lead to weight loss is unlikely to reverse type 2 diabetes. Even if you stop consuming glucose or starchy carbohydrates, your liver will continue to produce sugar from glycogen and from the byproducts of fats and proteins through a process called glyconeogenesis. The liver is the major chemical factory of the body, as I have said, and is responsible for the breakdown and synthesis of many chemicals or nutrients that the body needs or wants to eliminate as waste.[32]

Similarly, if you stop consuming fats without losing weight, you will not reverse type 2 diabetes. If you eat starchy carbs, they will be converted to sugar. Excess sugar will be stored, first in small amounts as glycogen, and second in unlimited amounts as fat. Thus, without eating fats, you end up making them from carbohydrates. Hence, type 2 diabetes can't be reversed by restricting fat or carbohydrate intake without weight loss.

Type 2 diabetes can't be reversed by restricting fat or carbohydrate intake without weight loss

Losing weight is an indication that you are burning or losing fat. It also indicates that you have switched from burning carbohydrates to fats. Burning fats improves insulin sensitivity and allows insulin to facilitate entry of sugar into the cells. This improves insulin sensitivity and reduces insulin resistance. In turn, sugar levels in blood fall because the cells are using the sugar to produce energy. This breaks down the chain of events caused by insulin resistance and improves other conditions, such as high blood pressure, blood clot formation, high cholesterol and inflammation.

Fats are initially broken down into ketones. Ketones are in turn broken down by a process called ketosis to produce fuel needed for body operations. Ketones are harmless and are flushed out of the body through urine or breath. Ketosis may produce bad breath, often called 'keto breath' characterised by a distinct taste or odour in the mouth. Some people describe the taste as metallic and that the odour is similar to the smell of nail polish. The smell can be reduced by drinking more water, sucking mints or chewing gum, or using a mouthwash.

Intermittent fasting is an easy way to lose weight, as I have described. It helps us reduce our total calorie intake because our stomach reduces in size when fasting so that we feel full easily when eating. In addition, intermittent fasting reduces levels of ghrelin, the hunger hormone, in our blood so that we don't feel that we are starving. A person who just reduces the amount of calories they consume without intermittent fasting will feel very hungry and this can be the cause of failure of calorie restriction plans.

As I have said, intermittent fasting has many other health benefits apart from weight loss, including reduction of blood pressure, increased insulin sensitivity, reduced inflammation, a decrease in LDL cholesterol, and a reduced risk of heart disease, blood clot formation, autoimmune diseases and cancers.

Be mindful of the quantity and quality of what you eat

While losing weight, you need to consider both the quantity and quality of your diet. Intermittent fasting helps you to significantly downsize your food intake, to below the recommended daily dietary requirements (2000 kcal per day for women and 2500 kcal for men). Calculating how many calories you have burnt and how many calories you have eaten may be difficult and impractical, as I have explained.

To overcome this difficulty, I recommend that you reduce your plate size and eat from smaller plates. Eat everything in smaller helpings than you used to. With intermittent fasting your stomach shrinks in size so that you start eating smaller meals than before. Intermittent fasting therefore helps you to downsize to a smaller plate without feeling that you are starving. Once you have established your new diet routine, you must stick to it and not go back to your previous way of eating. This is the only way you can sustain a healthy weight.

Some people think that reducing your food intake by half is not practical. It is feasible because, if you are obese or overweight, you must consistently be eating more than your body requires daily. There are people eating two or even three times the amount of food they need per day. Therefore, reducing your intake by half is completely doable. I reduced my food intake by 50% and lost 12.5% of my weight.

The second thing you should consider about your diet as you lose weight is the quality of what you eat. You are reducing the amount you eat for the long term. In fact, this is a lifelong change in diet. Therefore, you should make sure that your small plate is balanced. For normal, non-diabetic people, it is advisable that one third of our total food intake be made up of complex (not refined) starchy carbohydrates, another third of fruit and vegetables, and the last third of healthy oils and proteins. Complex starchy carbs, fruit and vegetables provide the fibre you need.

However, if you want to reverse diabetes, my experience is that you need to significantly reduce the amount of carbs/sugar you eat and either maintain or slightly reduce fat and protein. One study found that losing about 10 to 15 kg can reverse diabetes.[28] To reverse diabetes, instead of basing your diet on carbs as currently recommended by UK Eatwell guide, base your diet on protein and fat. Avoid sugar and refined carbohydrates. Even some fruits have lots of sugar and should be avoided. Do not reduce your intake of vegetables below the recommended daily intake because they provide essential minerals and vitamins.

Exercise complements intermittent fasting

Exercise is complementary to intermittent fasting in the treatment or reversal of type 2 diabetes. Exercise alone without weight loss is unlikely to succeed. When you exercise, you burn body fuel for energy. The primary body fuel burnt during exercise is glycogen which is easily converted to sugar for immediate energy. In the absence of sugar or glycogen, the body burns fats for energy.

Exercise can help you lose weight. However, the effect of exercise on weight loss is small. For example, you need to jog for one hour to burn 500 calories, which is equivalent to five slices of bread. Therefore, many people find it difficult to lose weight by simply doing exercise without a weight-loss dietary plan.

Second 20/80 rule: Type 2 diabetes is treated 80% by weight loss and 20% by exercise

Blood sugar drops with weight loss, but sometimes may remain borderline, fluctuating between normal and abnormal. I noticed that, when my weight loss was half way complete (5 kg lost), when I exercised, my blood sugar dropped to normal levels and when I failed to exercise it rose to abnormal levels. Exercise complements the effect of weight loss by removing any small excess sugar from the blood. It helps you to completely bring down your blood sugar levels so that you don't have to take pills. I estimate that my diabetes was reversed 80% by weight loss and 20% by exercise. I call this my *'second 20/80 rule'*.

Dietary fibre lowers blood sugar

Dietary fibre, or 'roughage', consists of complex carbohydrates obtained from plant-based food that our body can't digest. Unlike fats, carbs or proteins which are digested and absorbed, fibre is not digested by the bowel. Based on their relative solubility in water, dietary fibres can be classified as soluble and insoluble. The fact that dietary fibres are indigestible may sound as if fibre is purely a byproduct of digestion that is sent out as waste without any benefits to the body. However, the truth is completely the opposite. Insoluble fibres have the ability to bind to toxic chemicals, including carcinogens (cancer-causing chemicals) and mutagens (chemicals that cause genetic mutation) that are formed during the digestion of food and eliminate them in stool. Soluble fibres can be fermented in the large bowel to short-chain fatty acids that are a good, non-insulin-related source of energy.[33]

Most people are aware that dietary fibre is good for their health. They have been told that food rich in fibre reduces constipation. What many do not know is the wide range of health benefits associated with dietary fibre, or the types of dietary fibre.

Fibre, especially soluble fibre, slows the absorption of sugar and therefore reduces blood sugar levels

There are two types of dietary fibre – the soluble fibre which dissolves in water and the insoluble fibre which doesn't. Soluble fibre can be obtained from different food sources, including carrots, apples, oats, peas, barley, psyllium and citrus fruits. Insoluble fibre on the other hand can be obtained from whole grains, beans and vegetables including potatoes, green beans and cauliflower. Many fruits and vegetables contain both types of fibre. Understanding the different types of dietary fibre is important because they convey different benefits. In order to take advantage of the wide array of benefits, it is recommended to eat different types of foods that contain fibre. In fact, all plant-based foods contain fibre.

Refined food does not contain fibre because the fibre is removed during food processing. In fact, refined food promotes weight gain which can be counterproductive to any efforts to lose weight.

There are two hormones that regulate hunger and satiety, as I described earlier. Ghrelin, the hunger hormone, is produced by the stomach and increases your desire to eat. Leptin, the satiety hormone, is produced by fatty tissue and makes you feel full and satisfied. Refined foods impair ghrelin and leptin responses and cause people to overeat because they cannot recognise when they are full.

The health benefits of dietary fibre are many:
- Cholesterol (lowers blood cholesterol)
- Heart disease (lowers risk of heart disease)
- Intestines (promotes bowel health)
- Neoplasm (lowers risk of cancer)
- Obesity (promotes weight loss)
- Sugar (lowers blood sugar).

Soluble fibre lowers levels of low density lipoprotein (LDL) cholesterol and improves the cholesterol profile. It is therefore recommended that people with high LDL cholesterol and diabetes eat foods with high levels of soluble fibre, such as carrots, apples, oats, peas, barley, psyllium and citrus fruits.

High-fibre foods tend to contain fewer calories and fill the stomach and so you are likely to eat less. In addition, a high-fibre diet improves the ghrelin and leptin responses so that you can stay satisfied for longer. Overall, eating lots of fibre reduces calorie intake and contributes to weight loss.

High insoluble-fibre food normalises bowel movement by increasing the volume and weight of the stools. It also softens the stools and thereby reduces constipation. The fibre absorbs water and adds bulk to the stools making them much easier to pass.

Foods high in insoluble fibre reduce the risk of hemorrhoids and the development of small pouches in the bowel or colon called diverticular disease. Studies also show that a high-fibre diet reduces the risk of bowel cancer.[34] Indeed, a high-fibre diet is good for overall bowel health.

Fibre, especially soluble fibre, slows the absorption of sugar and therefore reduces blood sugar levels. It is therefore critical that people with diabetes have a high-fibre diet.

Finally, studies have shown that dietary fibre has health-related benefits for lowering high blood pressure, reducing inflammation and reducing the risk of dying from heart disease and all cancers.[35]

Practical tips for reversing type 2 diabetes

The acronym SAFEST (smoking, alcohol, food, exercise, stress and treatment) is used to manage sick fat disease in general. When it comes to type 2 diabetes specifically, the most important element is food (weight loss). Without significant weight loss, it is almost impossible to reverse type 2 diabetes.

The second aspect which is related to weight loss is to significantly reduce carbs/sugar intake. Most of the calorie reduction that leads to weight loss should come from carbs rather than protein and fat.

The third most important element in the reversal of diabetes is exercise. Type 2 diabetes can be reversed through the combination of weight loss by intermittent fasting and exercise. However, if you smoke, you will need to stop; if you drink alcohol, make sure that you moderate your intake. Extreme stress should also be recognised and correctly managed.

1. Intermittent fasting

Weight loss is at the heart of diabetic treatment and reversal, as I have explained. Aim to lose between 10 and 15% of your weight.

Chapter Six

You may need to lose up to 20% if your weight gain has gone to the extreme. Your BMI can serve as a guide, but having a normal BMI is not enough because it doesn't tell you where your body fat is located. Abdominal location of fat is more dangerous than lower body (thighs and hips).

In order to lose 12.5% of my weight, I reduced my energy/calorie intake by 50%. You too will need to significantly reduce your total calorie intake. As you reduce the amount you eat, make sure that your diet is balanced. Pay particular attention to fish, fibre and vegetables in your diet.

One of the easiest ways to lose weight is intermittent fasting. When you fast, you switch from burning sugar to burning fat and this helps you lose weight easily. Intermittent fasting also has many more benefits beyond weight loss.

2. Exercise

Exercise complements the effect of intermittent fasting. It contributes to weight loss, improves insulin sensitivity and enables you to finally quit pills and needles for diabetes.

Note that intermittent fasting has a far bigger effect on weight loss than exercise alone. Experts recommend that we undertake 150 to 300 minutes of moderate aerobic exercise (or 75 to 150 minutes of vigorous exercise) every week. Aerobic exercises include brisk walking, jogging, running, swimming and cycling. In order to reverse diabetes, you will need to top up weight loss with exercise. I recommend you do the exercise daily, rather than a few days a week. If your blood sugar level remains high or borderline, you either need to lose more weight or to increase the amount of exercise you do. You may need to do more exercise than the recommended 150 to 300 minutes per week. However, start small and increase progressively as you build confidence and physical endurance.

Strength training exercises such as squats, push-ups, lunges, bench press, weight lifting, plank, resistance banks and weight machines, help build your muscles. Bigger muscles increase sugar burning and insulin sensitivity, and help you to reverse diabetes.

3. Moderate alcohol use, quit smoking and manage stress

If you drink, moderate your alcohol use. Excessive alcohol intake will exacerbate diabetes by reducing sensitivity to insulin and/or causing chronic pancreatitis, although moderate intake seems to be protective against type 2 diabetes in both men and women.[36, 37] If you smoke, stop – smoking is a risk factor for type 2 diabetes because nicotine and other chemicals in cigarette smoke can reduce insulin sensitivity and can also cause mass dysfunction of pancreatic β-cells (the cells that produce insulin) and actual loss of β-cell mass.[38]

Exercise will also help in the management of extreme stress. Other stress management techniques, such as meditation, getting social support, smiling and laughing, and taking a break from particular stressors can also be of great help.

Diabetes during pregnancy

If you have diabetes, it's important to make sure that your blood sugar level is normal before getting pregnant and throughout pregnancy. If you develop diabetes during pregnancy (gestational diabetes), it's also important to ensure good blood sugar control.

Complications of diabetes to the baby include excessive weight gain, preterm birth, stillbirth, low blood sugar, serious breathing difficulty (respiratory distress syndrome) at birth, as well as obesity and type 2 diabetes later in life. Complications to the mother include high blood pressure during pregnancy (pre-eclampsia), surgical delivery (C-section), and future diabetes.

Chapter Six

Some women with gestational diabetes will respond to diet and exercise, but the majority will need medications such as oral sugar-lowering drugs or insulin injections to bring down their blood sugar level during pregnancy. It's recommended that women undertake 150 minutes of moderate intensity exercise per week during pregnancy and muscle strengthening activities twice a week.

The diet of a pregnant woman should be similar to a balanced diet for a non-pregnant woman. In addition, a pregnant woman may need iron and folic acid supplementation to prevent anaemia and birth defects.

Do not increase calories during pregnancy. It's only in the last three months of pregnancy that you will need an extra 200 calories per day. On the other hand, do not try to lose weight during pregnancy.

Gestational diabetes increases the risk of developing diabetes later in life, so it's important to embark on a lifestyle change after childbirth to prevent sick fat disease. Six weeks after childbirth, most women are physiologically ready to start exercise and weight loss plans.

Chapter Seven

High blood pressure

After trying different pill-free treatment plans for high blood pressure, the only thing that finally worked for me was daily moderate to vigorous intensity exercise.

> **Lesson 7**
>
> High blood pressure is a disease caused by a sedentary lifestyle; the cornerstone of its reversal or prevention is physical activity.

Finding a cure for high blood pressure was a daunting task. I tried out 70 things and almost gave up. For over five years, I kept trying. Inwardly, I believed there was something I could do to stop having to take pills for this condition.

The last thing that I tried was exercise. I jogged and ran every morning for one hour for a month. One month of regular moderate to vigorous intensity exercise was not enough to reverse my high blood pressure. I continued with jogging and running every morning for six months. After six months of moderate to vigorous intensity exercise, my blood pressure dropped to very low levels that I had never seen before. I stopped antihypertensive pills and continued with my morning workouts.

A daily workout of 60 minutes or more can reverse your high blood pressure provided you continue for about six months – don't give up!

I discovered the cure for high blood pressure by accident because I didn't continue the workout for six months with the hope that it would have this effect. I continued because it made me feel healthier and stronger.

I learnt that working out could reverse high blood pressure provided you continue for a long time. Working out strengthens your heart muscles to pump blood better, and time is needed for this to happen. Exercise is the centerpiece for reversing high blood pressure. A daily workout of 60 minutes or more can reverse your high blood pressure provided you continue for about six months.

There is a lot of information out there about high blood pressure. The difficulty is separating facts from myths and misconceptions. Many of these sources treat every fact as if they are of equal importance. In this book, I distinguish exercise from other things which are helpful but do not have the same level of importance if you want to reverse high blood pressure. From my experience as a patient, there are four important points that everyone should know about high blood pressure.

- Physical inactivity causes high blood pressure
- Exercise is the cornerstone of reversal of high blood pressure
- Weight loss complements exercise
- Alcohol, smoking and stress reduction also help.

Physical inactivity causes high blood pressure

An ideal blood pressure (BP) is considered to be between 90/60 and 120/80 mm Hg. The upper number (90 or 120) is called the systolic BP and measures the force at which the heart pumps blood around the body. The lower number (60 or 80) is the diastolic BP and is a measure of the resistance to the blood flow in the blood vessels. A BP of 140/90 mm Hg and higher is considered high. A BP of between 120/80 mm Hg and 140/90 mm Hg could mean either you have high blood pressure or you are at risk of developing it. Everyone's BP will be slightly different and so what is considered high for one person may be normal for another.

High blood pressure seen in sick fat disease is caused by either of two systems – the renin-angiotensin system (RAS) or the sympathetic nervous system (SNS).

1. Renin–angiotensin system (RAS)

The renin–angiotensin system (RAS) is a 'key worker system' that regulates our blood pressure. Its activation causes our blood pressure to increase. Hormones are chemical messengers that are our body's 'key workers'. Sick fat disease inappropriately activates the renin-angiotensin system. Once activated, the system fires signals that cause a metabolic cascade which leads to the production of a hormone called angiotensin II by the kidneys. Angiotensin II causes the blood vessels to tighten up, squeezing the blood, which in turn raises the BP.

Aldosterone causes the kidneys to retain sodium and flush out potassium. Sodium retention raises blood pressure

Angiotensin II also causes the production of another hormone called aldosterone by the adrenal gland. Aldosterone causes the kidneys to retain sodium and flush out potassium. Sodium retention raises blood pressure. Some medicines for high blood pressure, such as captopril and ramipril, work by blocking the renin-angiotensin mechanism.

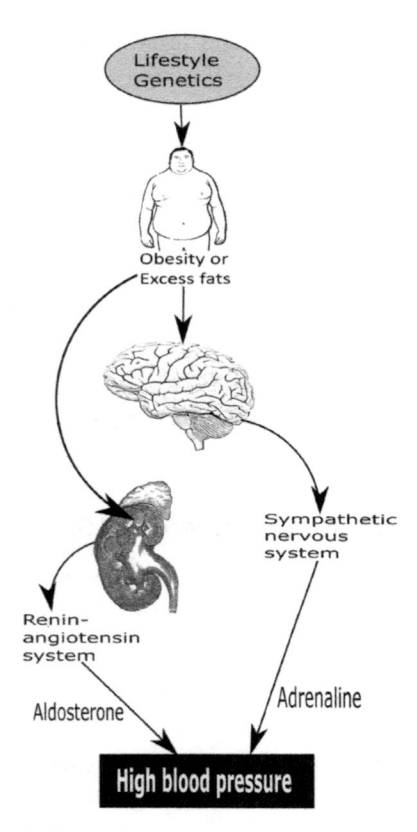

Figure 12: How high blood pressure develops

2. Sympathetic nervous system (SNS)

The sympathetic nervous system (SNS) is one of the two main divisions of the autonomic nervous system (the other being the parasympathetic nervous system – PNS) that is responsible for our 'fight or flight' response among other things.

The autonomic nervous system is a control system that acts largely unconsciously and regulates bodily functions, such as heart rate, digestion, respiratory rate, pupillary response in the eyes, urination, and sexual arousal. The SNS prepares the body for the 'fight or flight' response during any potential danger. The PNS, on the other hand, inhibits the body from overworking and restores it to a calm and composed state. SNS activation causes BP to rise. Once activated, the system fires electrical signals that lead to the release of the hormone adrenaline by the adrenal gland.

Imagine that you are in a room next to a zoo and suddenly a lion gets into the room. You don't have time to think. Your body's sympathetic nervous system triggers the immediate release of adrenaline that increases your heart rate, breathing, blood flow to your muscles, sweating and blood pressure. The high blood pressure is caused by the narrowing of blood vessels and increased blood flow.

If the lion is caught by the zoo guards, these responses will normally subside, the blood vessels will relax and your body will go back to normal.

Adrenaline increases your heart rate, breathing, blood flow to your muscles, sweating and blood pressure

However, with sick fat disease there is sustained firing by the sympathetic nervous system. The blood vessels remain permanently narrowed and high blood pressure is prolonged.

Some medicines for high blood pressure, such as clonidine and methyldopa, act by blocking the sympathetic nervous system which in turn causes the blood vessels to widen.

Exercise is the cornerstone of reversal of high blood pressure

Exercise is central to the treatment of high blood pressure. While it may not have a significant effect on weight loss, it does have a big impact on blood pressure by blocking the two mechanisms responsible for high blood pressure seen in sick fat disease:

1. First, exercise blocks the renin-angiotensin system (RAS) described above. This causes the blood vessels to widen and the kidneys to flush out sodium. These two actions reduce blood pressure.
2. Second, exercise blocks the sympathetic nervous system (SNS). This causes the blood vessels to relax and widen which in turn reduces the blood pressure.

Exercise blocks the two mechanisms responsible for high blood pressure seen in sick fat disease

In addition, sweating (caused by exercise or warm weather) lowers blood pressure by causing the dilation of blood vessels under the skin as well as loss of water and salt. Sweating is a natural method the body uses to control body temperature. When your body starts to heat up, whether because of exercise or outside temperature, it releases sweat from the more than 2-4 million eccrine glands spread out across your skin, pouring liquid through pores to lower body temperature. Sweating induces a 'diuretic' effect by causing increased loss of salt, including sodium, and this lowers blood pressure.[38a]

From my experience, the effect of exercise on blood pressure is far more than the effect of weight loss. However, the effect is not immediate. You will need to undertake moderate to vigorous intensity exercise for about six months before you can start reaping the benefits.

Aerobic or 'cardio' exercises cause repetitive contraction of large muscle groups which in turn forces the heart to work hard and pump blood to the muscles. Regular 'cardio' workouts, such as jogging, brisk walking, running, cycling, swimming, yoga, dancing, football, golf, hiking and basketball, increase the heart rate and train the heart muscles. You need to train your heart muscles to pump blood more efficiently and this takes time. The longer the duration of each exercise, the better the results. Cardio training over several months causes a significant fall in blood pressure.

Experts recommend that people undertake at least 150 to 300 minutes of moderate intensity exercise or 75 to 150 minutes of vigorous intensity exercise per week. For 'cardio' training to treat or reverse high blood pressure, *I recommend that you do 60 minutes or more of moderate to vigorous exercise per day for six months*. Better results are obtained with vigorous than with moderate intensity exercise; so the higher the intensity the better.

I found that sweat-inducing exercises are more effective than exercises that do not cause sweating. I have found my systolic blood pressure to be 10 to 20 mm Hg lower and my diastolic blood pressure to be 5 to 10 mm Hg lower when I sweat than when I don't after exercise. The higher the sweating, the lower the blood pressure. During winter, I often wear something warm during exercise to induce sweating. Numerous studies have found a correlation between temperature and blood pressure and have also generally shown higher blood pressure during winter. The explanation is that cold weather activates both the sympathetic nervous system and the renin–angiotensin system. Warm weather does the reverse as well as inducing sweating.[38a]

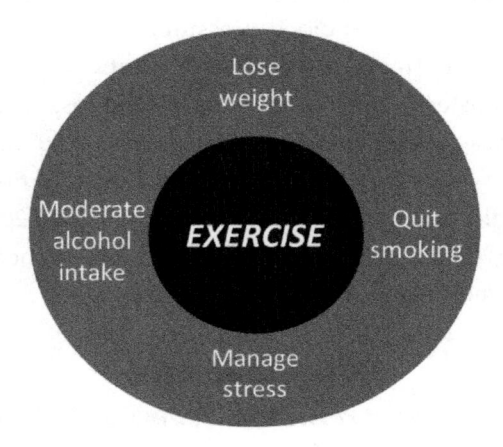

Figure 13: Exercise is the cornerstone of hypertension reversal

Continue to exercise after stopping your BP pills to prevent recurrence of high blood pressure. The exercise must be one that increases your heart beat or causes you to sweat. Low intensity exercise has little effect on blood pressure. Blood pressure drops and is lowest immediately after each moderate to vigorous intensity exercise.

I was able to lower my blood pressure by undertaking 60 minutes of jogging and/or running every day for six months. After six months I found that my blood pressure had dropped so significantly that I didn't need any antihypertensive medicines anymore. I believe I could have stopped the medication even earlier, but since I wasn't taking my BP regularly I didn't know that it had dropped significantly until I took it after six months of exercise.

Weight loss complements exercise

Weight is important if you want to say 'goodbye' to your antihypertensive pills. Studies have shown that by losing 5 kg (8.8 pounds), your systolic and diastolic blood pressure can drop by 4.5 to 3.2 mm Hg respectively.[39] If you have mild high blood pressure, weight loss alone can be sufficient to control it.

Weight loss improves blood pressure, although exercise has a greater impact. This is the reverse of what I found for type 2 diabetes. Diabetes is affected more by weight loss than by exercise. In my case, I estimate that my BP was treated 80% by exercise and 20% by weight loss (my third 20/80 rule) and my diabetes 80% by weight loss and 20% by exercise (my second 20/80 rule – page 89). My first 20/80 rule states that 80% of weight loss is due to reducing food intake and 20% to exercise.

Third 20/80 rule:
High blood pressure is reversed 80% by exercise and 20% by weight loss

Chapter Seven

Practical tips to reverse high blood pressure

Sick fat disease in general can be managed using the acronym SAFEST (smoking, alcohol, food, exercise, stress and treatment). The cornerstone of reversing high blood pressure is exercise. Without adequate physical activity, it is almost impossible to reverse high blood pressure.

The two most important elements are exercise and food (weight loss). The other elements (alcohol, smoking and stress) should also be taken into account if they are found to be major contributors to the high blood pressure.

1. Exercise

As I have said, exercise is the centerpiece for reversal of high BP. Experts recommend 150 to 300 minutes of moderate exercise (or 75 to 150 minutes of vigorous exercise) per week for everyone. However, if you are treating high BP and want to stop taking pills, you may need more exercise than recommended for the general public. *I recommend that you aim to do 60 minutes or more of moderate to vigorous sweat-inducing exercise per day for about six months.* You will obtain better results with vigorous compared to moderate intensity exercises. Once high BP is reversed, you need to continue with your exercise to ensure that it remains low.

2. Weight loss

Weight loss complements the effect of exercise on BP. It is estimated that for every 1 kg of weight loss, there is a reduction of 1 mm Hg of systolic BP. Use intermittent fasting to help you lose weight easily.

3. Quit smoking, moderate alcohol use and manage stress

In addition to exercise and weight loss, quit smoking if you smoke, moderate alcohol intake if you drink and correctly manage stress. Stress raises BP and failure to manage stress can be one of the reasons your BP remains high. Exercise helps in stress management. You can also make use of other stress management techniques such as meditation and social support (see Chapter 11).

High blood pressure during pregnancy

If you have high blood pressure before pregnancy (chronic hypertension) or you develop high blood pressure during pregnancy (gestational hypertension), make sure that you follow your doctor's advice and treatment to prevent the risk of complications. Complications include seizures in the mother (eclampsia), stroke, kidney failure, blood clotting problems, preterm birth, surgical delivery (C-section) and premature detachment of the placenta from the uterine walls (placental abruption).

While taking your medication, you should do 150 minutes of moderate intensity exercise per week unless your doctor advises otherwise. Do not attempt to diet or lose weight during pregnancy or until six weeks after childbirth. Ensure you have a healthy nutritious diet.

Women who develop high blood pressure during pregnancy have a three to four times increased risk of developing high blood pressure in their lifetime and twice the risk of heart disease and stroke. Therefore, if you have had high blood pressure during pregnancy, it's important to adopt a healthy lifestyle to prevent complications in the future. These lifestyle changes include – as this book demonstrates – adequate exercise, healthy diet and healthy weight.

Chapter Eight

Exercise

I changed my desk from a sitting to a standing work station. That brought my blood pressure below what I was able to achieve with exercise alone.

> **Lesson 8**
>
> While regular exercise is important for good health, better results are obtained when you stay physically active throughout the day.

I was curious and eager to know more about myself and my health. When I discovered that exercise was the ultimate cure for high blood pressure, I didn't stop there. I decided to find out what will happen if one was physically active throughout the day. I noticed that, each day I came back from work, I did between 1000 and 2000 steps. I spent most of the time sitting. In the morning before going to work, my workout yielded up to 10,000 steps.

In order to stay physically active throughout the day, I changed my desk to a standing work station. I remained standing while working, reading emails and writing, and held standing meetings. Instead of using the lift, I used the staircase. The number of my steps during the day increased from 1000–2000 to 4000–5000 (excluding the 10,000 steps due to working out).

Before the standing work station, my BP was lowest after the morning workout and tended to rise gradually during the day. The rise in BP was more with the systolic than the diastolic BP. The systolic BP tended to rise by about 10 to 20 mm Hg during the day. By staying active throughout the day, I noticed that the systolic BP was 10 mm Hg lower during the day than it would otherwise be when I wasn't physically active.

I therefore concluded that while regular exercise is important for good health, it's even better to stay physically active throughout the day and between the exercises.

The following are major points about physical activity that everyone needs to know:
- Our ancestors burnt more calories than we do
- Aerobic exercises prevent heart disease
- Moderate and vigorous intensity exercises yield better results than low intensity
- The amount of exercise required varies with age and ability
- We should stay physically active throughout the day
- Physical inactivity is extremely harmful to your health.

Our ancestors burnt more calories than we do

Human beings have lived on earth for at least two millions years. During the prehistoric period, people were nomads and survived by hunting and gathering food. At this time, people burnt more calories per day than we do today.

During the agricultural period, starting approximately 10,000 years ago, nomadic hunting and gathering societies were replaced by agricultural societies in which people grew their own food and domesticated animals. Despite this change, people remained physically very active and expended more calories than today because everything was done manually.

Chapter Eight

The industrial period, from the mid-18th century to the end of the Second World War (1945), saw the development of the steam engine and electrically powered machines. Many people moved from farms to cities and joined the industrial workforce. Despite the fact that steam engine and electrical power were increasingly being used, a majority of people walked to work, climbed stairs and did a lot of physically demanding jobs every day.

Our evolutionary history has prepared humankind for one life, and yet we have decided to live another

During the technological period following the Second World War, there was a rapid growth of energy-saving devices both at home and in the workplace. People now go to work by car instead of walking, use lifts instead of stairs, use machines to do the work for them and sit all day long on the computer at work and watching television at home. This means that today human beings burn far fewer calories per day than their ancestors.

The evolutionary history has prepared mankind for one life, and yet we have decided to live another. This shift in calorie expenditure has significant implications for the disease patterns we see today. Sick fat disease has become a pandemic. Obesity, high blood pressure, type 2 diabetes and heart disease have become commonplace. We still have a few nomadic communities in the world today. These nomadic groups continue to expend more calories per day, show higher level of physical fitness and seem to be spared the 'chronic' diseases that the whole world is suffering from due to a sedentary lifestyle.

Aerobic exercises prevent heart disease

Four types of exercise are good for your health. Each type has its specific health benefits. The four types are: aerobic, strength building, stretching and balance exercises.

1. Aerobic exercises

Aerobic exercises lower blood pressure, prevent heart disease and prevent or treat sick fat disease as a whole. 'Aerobic' can be used to describe any exercise that increases your heart rate and breathing. It forces the heart and lungs to work more. Such exercise trains the heart and lungs and increases endurance. Aerobic exercises are also called 'cardio' exercises.

Aerobic exercises burn body fat, relax blood vessels, reduce blood pressure, reduce inflammation, boost mood and lower LDL cholesterol

Aerobic exercises burn body fat, relax blood vessels, reduce blood pressure, reduce inflammation, boost mood, raise HDL cholesterol and lower LDL cholesterol. Over the long term, aerobic exercises make the heart stronger, and reduce the risk of stroke, high blood pressure, type 2 diabetes, heart disease, depression, falls, breast cancer and colon cancer.

Examples of aerobic exercises include brisk walking, jogging, running, swimming, biking, digging, hoeing, dancing, football, tennis and other sports. It's recommended that you do 150 to 300 minutes of moderate intensity aerobic exercise per week.

2. Strength training

Strength training builds muscles, makes us stronger and gives us a better body configuration. This is particularly important because we lose muscle mass as we get older. As we lose muscle mass, we become weaker, our bones weaken, and we can easily lose our posture and balance. Strength training does not only build the muscles – it stimulates bone growth, helps control weight, improves posture and balance, reduces stress, reduces pain in the joints and lower back, and lowers blood sugar because the increased muscle mass uses more sugar.

Strength building exercises are also called resistance training exercises. They include squats, push-ups, lunges, bench presses, weight lifting, plank, resistance banks and weight machines. Two or three sessions of strength building exercises per week will keep you in good health.

When you exercise regularly, your muscles need more blood, and in response to regular exercise, muscles grow more blood vessels by expanding the network of capillaries (the smallest blood vessels) that feed them. In addition, muscle cells increase the levels of the enzymes that allow them to use oxygen to generate energy. As a result, you get more oxygen-rich blood and a more efficient metabolism. This explains why people who exercise regularly develop endurance and strength.

As we get older, we are much more vulnerable to calcium and vitamin D deficiency. This is because with age we have reduced intestinal absorption of calcium, decreased capacity of the skin to synthesise vitamin D and reduced efficiency of the kidneys to retain vitamin D or convert vitamin D into the most active form required by the body. Deficiency in calcium and vitamin D makes bones weak and susceptible to fractures. Therefore, in order to boost your bone health and strength, make sure you eat calcium and vitamin D rich foods, such as green leafy vegetables, milk and dairy products and sardines.

3. *Stretching*

Stretching or flexibility exercises help maintain flexibility. As we grow older, we lose flexibility in our muscles and tendons. The muscles shorten and don't function so well. This increases the risk of muscle cramps and pains, strains, joint pain, muscle and tendon damage, falling, fractures and being unable to go through our routine activities. Therefore, it is important that we ensure that we remain flexible especially as we get older.

Examples of stretching exercises include arm circles, matching in place, hip circles, shoulder rolls, arm stretches, anterior and posterior shoulder stretches and forward and lateral leg swings. Stretching exercises should be done on a daily basis.

4. Balance exercises

As we get older, the system that maintains our posture and balance starts to break down. This system includes our leg muscles and joints, our inner ears and our vision. Balance exercises help delay or repair the breakdown of our system in charge of balance, make us feel steadier on our feet and prevent falls and are especially important if you have had a fall or a near-fall or you fear that you will fall.

Examples of balance exercise include yoga, tai chi, standing on one foot with eyes open or closed, heel-to-toe inline walks with eyes open or closed, and strengthening leg muscles through exercises such as squats and leg lifts.

Moderate and vigorous intensity exercises yield better results

There are three types of exercise according to intensity: low intensity, moderate intensity and vigorous exercise. Moderate and vigorous intensity exercises are better for your health compared with low intensity exercises such as walking.

1. Low intensity exercise

Low intensity exercise is defined as an exercise in which you don't feel you are exerting yourself. It includes normal walking and other movements which do not increase your heart rate or breathing. Low intensity exercises are not 'cardio' exercises and have little effect on your heart. Although they are not specifically beneficial for the heart, they do provide general health benefits that vary depending on the type. It is recommended that between taking moderate to vigorous exercise, you stay active by undertaking repetitive low intensity exercise such as walking and standing up while working.

2. Moderate intensity exercise

Moderate intensity exercises are exercises during which you can talk comfortably but can't sing. They increase your heart rate and breathing and have numerous health benefits. Examples of moderate intensity exercises include brisk walking, jogging, water aerobics, gardening, dancing, tennis (doubles) and biking more slowly than 10 miles per hour.

3. Vigorous or intense exercise

Vigorous exercises are those exercises during which you can say a few words but not a full sentence. Like the moderate intensity exercises, vigorous exercises increase your heart rate and breathing and are good for your heart. They also have a wide range of health benefits. The benefit from one minute of vigorous exercise is roughly equivalent to two minutes of moderate exercise. Examples of vigorous intensity exercises include hiking uphill or with a heavy backpack, running, swimming, tennis (singles), cycling 10 miles per hour or more, jumping rope, aerobic dancing and heavy gardening like continuous digging or hoeing.

The amount of exercise required varies with age and ability

The type of exercise and how long you do it for depend on your age. The risk of adverse events from exercise is relatively low, and the health benefits accrued from such activity outweigh the risks. Children tend to be more physically active than adults.

- Toddlers (1 to 2 years): At least 180 minutes (3 hours) of a variety of physical activity of any intensity per day.
- Preschool age (3 to 4 years): At least 180 minutes (3 hours) of a variety of physical activies per day. The 180 minutes should include 60 minutes of moderate to vigorous intensity physical activity.
- Children and young people (5 to 18 years): It is recommended they undertake moderate to vigorous exercise for 60 minutes every day. This should include strength training exercise to build muscles and bones three times per week.
- Adults (19 to 64 years): Adults should undertake at least 150 minutes of moderate intensity exercise or 75 minutes of vigorous exercise per week. This should include a combination of aerobic and strength-training exercise.
- Older adults (65 years and above): Older adults should aim to do 150 minutes of moderate intensity (or 75 minutes of vigorous) exercise per week. They should also add stretching and balance exercises.
- Pregnant women: Pregnant women should undertake 150 minutes of moderate intensity aerobic exercises per week. They should also do muscle-strengthening activities twice a week. Exercise in pregnancy helps control weight gain and reduce high blood pressure problems, prevents 'gestational' diabetes, and improves fitness, mood and sleep.
- Reversing high blood pressure: Adults with high blood pressure need more exercise to lower their blood pressure and go medication-free. I recommend 60 minutes or more per day of sweat-inducing moderate to vigorous intensity exercise if you want to reverse your high blood pressure. The higher the intensity of the exercise, the better. You should continue for about six months to start seeing results. Continue with this level of exercise even after you have gone pill-free.

Chapter Eight

Stay physically active throughout the day

It is important that between periods of deliberately exercising we stay physically active. Physical activity is often used to mean exercise. However, the two terms are not exactly the same. Physical activity refers to any bodily movement that leads to expenditure of energy. Physical activity includes exercise. Exercise is a type of structured activity that is specifically planned to develop and maintain physical fitness.

In the prehistoric era, physical activity was for hunting and food gathering. Although it contributed to health and fitness, it wasn't designed to maintain physical fitness. Our ancestors where physically active, but not through exercising. The concept of exercise came about when our lifestyle became sedentary. To maintain health and fitness, human beings came up with the notion of a structured physical activity called exercise. Exercise is an innovation to respond to our changing lifestyles. People now go to gyms and parks to exercise, while our ancestors didn't have such facilities – they had the jungles, forests and farms.

It is important that we shouldn't be fooled into believing that exercise is all the physical activity we need to do. We need to remain physically active between exercises and throughout the day. Staying physically active complements and boosts the benefits of exercising. I observed an additional drop in my blood pressure when I decided to change my sitting desk to a standing work station. By standing while working, I stayed physically active throughout the day. There are many other things you can do to shift from sitting to being active. For example, you can watch television while standing or while strolling round the room.

Physical inactivity is extremely harmful to your health

Exercising has many health benefits that go far beyond sick fat disease. Exercise reduces the risk of sick fat disease ABCD

(**A**bdominal obesity, **B**lood pressure, **C**holesterol and **D**iabetes). Sick fat disease increases your risk of heart disease and stroke.

In addition to sick fat disease, physical inactivity increases your risk for other health conditions which you can again use the acronym ABCD to remember:

A = Anxiety (plus stress and depression)
B = Bones
C = Cancers
D = Dementia (including Alzheimer's disease)

BRAIN
Reduced risk of depression, anxiety, and dementia

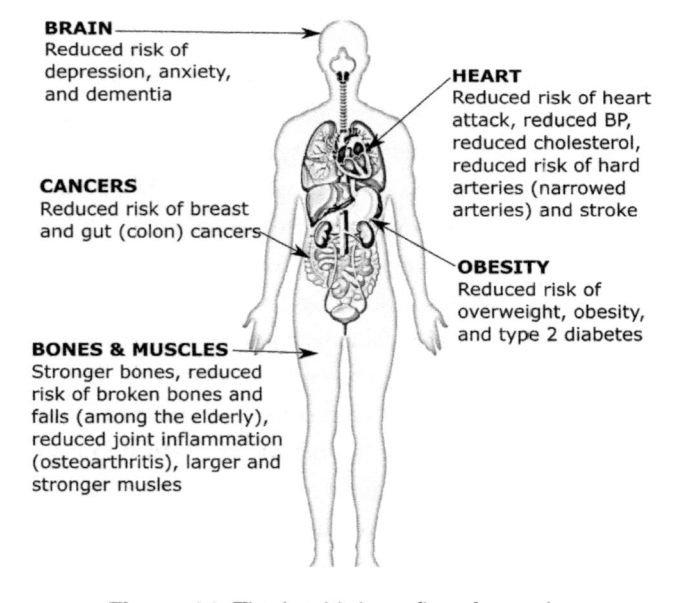

HEART
Reduced risk of heart attack, reduced BP, reduced cholesterol, reduced risk of hard arteries (narrowed arteries) and stroke

CANCERS
Reduced risk of breast and gut (colon) cancers

OBESITY
Reduced risk of overweight, obesity, and type 2 diabetes

BONES & MUSCLES
Stronger bones, reduced risk of broken bones and falls (among the elderly), reduced joint inflammation (osteoarthritis), larger and stronger musles

Figure 14: The health benefits of exercise

Physical activity and exercise provide enormous health benefits while inactivity does exactly the opposite. Sedentary lifestyle increases the risk of sick fat disease (obesity, high blood pressure, high cholesterol, type 2 diabetes, stroke, heart disease), brain diseases (anxiety, depression, stress, dementia, Alzheimer's disease), cancers (breast and bowel) and diseases of bones and muscles (weak bones, inflamed joints, loss of muscle mass).

Watching television, sitting or riding in cars contribute to overweight, obesity, heart disease, diabetes, high blood pressure and other chronic disease conditions. Exercise reduces the risk of heart disease and stroke by 35%, type 2 diabetes by 50%, breast cancer by 20%, early death by 30%, osteoarthritis by 83%, hip fracture by 68%, falls among the elderly by 30%, depression by 30% and dementia by 30%.

The health cost of physical inactivity

1. **Sick fat disease (ABCD)**
   A = Abdominal obesity
   B = Blood pressure (high)
   C = Cholesterol (high)
   D = Diabetes type 2

2. **Other inactivity-related health conditions (ABCD)**
   A = Anxiety (plus stress and depression)
   B = Bone problems
   C = Cancer
   D = Dementia (including Alzheimer's disease)

Chapter Nine

Drinking alcohol

I have a friend who had a car accident, was kidnapped and lost his job, all in one year. He started drinking heavily and became an alcoholic. All his life dreams were shattered.

> **Lesson 9**
>
> Deficient coping skills to deal with stressful life events can lead you to adopt unhealthy behaviours that become hard to break.

One of my friends went through the worst moments of his life went he was in his mid-thirties. Three stressful life events happened to him in one year. First, he had a car accident and knocked down a woman. Fortunately, there were no casualties. Nevertheless, the case went to court and his insurance company paid the damages. Second, he travelled abroad for a holiday and was kidnapped. The kidnappers asked for a ransom which his family paid before he was released. Third, he was fired from his job which was the main source of income for his family.

It took him six months to find another job. By the time he got that second job, he had started drinking heavily. He drank every day and came back home already drunk. He had become an alcoholic.

Before becoming an alcoholic, he had very positive plans for the future and was enthusiastic about them. He pursued his dreams with passion. When he became a drunk, he lost interest in everything. including his dreams. He was fired from his second job after working for just a year. He got a third job but then resigned after six months.

I learnt a lot from what he went through. It can be very tempting to use alcohol to help you forget about a stressful life event. Some people when going through difficult times, drink to get drunk. They drink heavily and quickly. They binge drink. Alcohol causes both excitement and depression. It can relax you immediately but after a few hours you get depressed. Heavy drinking can be difficult to stop even after the stressful life event is long gone.

> *Alcohol causes both excitement and depression. It can relax you immediately but after a few hours you get depressed*

Having learnt from my friend, I became very conscious about the risks of alcohol. As an adult, I drank wine and beer occasionally and in moderation. When I was diagnosed with diabetes and high blood pressure, I decided to check the effect of alcohol on my BP. I abstained from alcohol for six months and my BP didn't change. That was probably because I hadn't been drinking heavily. Heavy alcohol intake can raise BP significantly and can cause sick fat disease.

I did an internet search for 'alcohol' and got 1.15 billion hits. There are lots of facts, myths, misconceptions, misleading claims and even disagreements between experts. This chapter focuses on facts based on the latest scientific evidence. The facts are grouped under four major headings:
- The risks of drinking outweigh the benefits
- Heavy drinking increases the risk of sick fat disease

Chapter Nine

- Drinking during pregnancy can harm your baby
- There is no general consensus on the 'low risk limit'.

The risks of drinking outweigh the benefits

You may have come across many articles on the health benefits of drinking wine. The story started in the early 1990s, when the World Health Organization's MONICA Project revealed that, despite the high consumption of saturated fats in France, there was a low rate of heart disease. Scientists explained this 'French Paradox' by the fact that consumption of wine by the French was protective to their hearts. The explanation was plausible because low-to-moderate alcohol intake increases HDL cholesterol (see page 124) and reduces LDL cholesterol. Having a high level of HDL cholesterol is associated with a reduced risk of heart disease and stroke.

Emerging scientific evidence shows that the evidence from past studies on the benefits of alcohol may have been exaggerated

Between the 1990s and today more research has revealed many things that were not known in the 1990s. The Risk Threshold Study conducted across 19 high-income countries and published in the *Lancet* in 2018 provides us with more evidence. It was a huge study that included almost 600,000 drinkers. It showed that people who drank more than 100 g, or 12.5 units, of alcohol per week (equivalent to 5 to 6 standard glasses of wine or pints of beer) were likely to die sooner than those who drank no more than this amount.[40] Meanwhile, emerging scientific evidence shows that the evidence from past studies on the benefits of alcohol may have been exaggerated.

Heavy consumption of alcohol has both short-term and long-term effects and can lead to alcohol poisoning (as in binge drinking).

Short-term effects of alcohol

The short-term effects of alcohol can be either mild or severe depending on the amount the person has drunk. Short-term harmful consequences include loss of coordination, mood swings, excitement, relaxation, raised blood pressure, passing out, reduced body temperature, difficulty concentrating, poor judgement, vomiting, blurred or double vision, slow reaction times and many more.

Alcohol poisoning

Binge drinking can lead to alcohol poisoning. When we drink, the liver, which is our body's 'chemical factory', breaks down the alcohol and removes it from the body. The liver takes about one hour to break down one unit (8 g) of alcohol. One unit of alcohol is equivalent to half a standard glass of 12%-strength wine (one-third of a large glass of wine) or half a pint of 3.6% alcohol beer (one-third of a pint of 5.2% beer).

Drinking 8 units of alcohol for men (or 6 units of alcohol for women) in a single session is considered binge drinking

Binge drinking occurs when someone drinks a lot of alcohol in a short space of time or when they drink to get drunk. Drinking 8 units of alcohol for men (or 6 units of alcohol for women) in a single session is considered binge drinking.

Alcohol poisoning from binge drinking can lead to nausea, vomiting, confusion, slowed or irregular breathing, pale skin, blue-tinted skin, low body temperature (hypothermia), unconsciousness and seizures. Alcohol poisoning can cause permanent brain damage and even death.

Chapter Nine

Long-term effects of alcohol

Chronic heavy drinking is associated with serious health problems. Long-term harmful consequences include:
- Sick fat disease (high blood pressure, obesity, diabetes and high cholesterol which can lead to heart disease and stroke)
- Nutrient deficiencies (malnutrition, anaemia, calcium deficiency)
- Pregnancy problems (erectile dysfunction, irregular menstruation, miscarriage, stillbirth, foetal malformation)
- Cancers (mouth and throat, oesophageal, liver, breast, bowel)
- Liver disease (cirrhosis, fatty liver, hepatitis) and pancreatic disease (pancreatitis)
- Brain problems (memory loss, impaired coordination, impaired concentration, anxiety, alterations in mood, loss of attention span, trouble learning, depression, sleep changes, schizophrenia).

BRAIN
Loss of memory, loss of attention span, trouble learning, depression, anxiety, irritability, cravings, panic, sleeplessness, mood swings

LIVER
Scarring (cirrhosis)

PREGNANCY
Erectile dysfunction, irregular menstruation, stillbirths, miscarriages, malformed babies

HEART
High blood pressure, High cholesterol, Heart attack, Stroke

PANCREAS
Inflammation (pancreatitis)

GUT (DIGESTIVE)
Malnutrition, anaemia, calcium deficiency

CANCERS
Mouth, throat, liver, breast, bowel

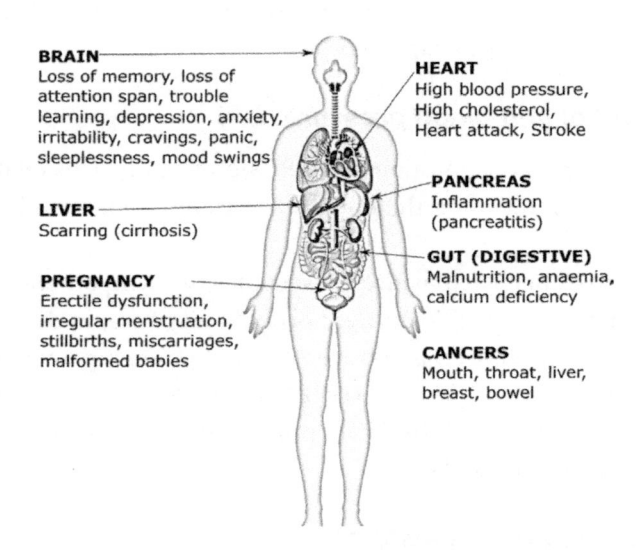

Figure 15: The harmful effects of alcohol

Several mental illnesses, including depression, stress, anxiety and schizophrenia, may cause people to drink too much. In these cases, alcohol is used as a self-medicating substance because of its relaxing and stimulating effects. However, the excitement induced by alcohol is short-lived and is followed by depression. The person is locked into a vicious cycle of depression-drinking-excitement-depression.

Heavy drinking increases the risk of sick fat disease

Heavy drinking can cause sick fat disease (obesity, high blood pressure, high cholesterol and diabetes).

1. Alcohol and obesity

Heavy alcohol use can lead to weight gain because alcohol carries higher calories (7.1 kcal/g) than carbohydrates (4 kcal/g) and protein (4 kcal/g). For this reason, those who drink heavily often develop apple-shaped obesity.

2. Alcohol and blood pressure (BP)

Heavy alcohol consumption raises BP significantly. This relationship is linear, meaning the higher the alcohol intake the higher the BP.

Scientists believe that alcohol activates the sympathetic nervous system (responsible for fight or flight response, as described earlier) which causes blood vessels to tighten up (contract), squeezing the blood. This causes BP to rise. Alcohol also increases the force with which the heart pumps blood round the body, which can also raise the BP.

3. Alcohol and cholesterol

Low-to-moderate use of alcohol increases levels of HDL cholesterol and reduces those of LDL cholesterol. The mechanism of action of moderate alcohol intake is still poorly understood, but studies suggest that alcohol affects the transport of cholesterol by increasing the liver's production of apoliprotein and lipoprotein particles (whose primary role is to transport lipids), decreases removal of circulating HDL, reduces synthesis of LDL and increases synthesis of HDL by regulating gene expression.[41] HDL cholesterol is associated with a reduced risk of heart disease and stroke.

However, with heavy drinking this benefit disappears completely. In fact, drinking more than 12.5 units or 100 g of alcohol per week increases the risk of heart disease and stroke.

Alcohol and diabetes

There are at least three ways that heavy alcohol consumption can cause diabetes. First, alcohol has lots of calories and heavy drinking can consequently cause obesity which is responsible for type 2 diabetes. Second, heavy drinking causes insulin resistance, a situation where insulin is unable to deliver sugar into the cells, as we have seen (Chapter 6). Third, heavy drinking also causes inflammation of the pancreas (pancreatitis). The pancreas is the organ that produces insulin and insulin lowers blood sugar as we have seen. The inflamed pancreas doesn't function normally and this can lead to diabetes.

Drinking alcohol during pregnancy can harm your baby

Women who drink alcohol while pregnant are at increased risk of miscarriage, stillbirth and foetal alcohol spectrum disorder (FASD), which is a name for various health, behaviour and learning problems that can affect babies if their mother drinks alcohol in pregnancy. Foetal alcohol syndrome is a type of FASD where the baby presents with brain damage and growth problems. A

baby with foetal alcohol spectrum disorder FASD might have any of the following:
- Low body weight
- Small head size
- Poor growth (smaller and shorter than average)
- Hyperactive behaviour
- Poor memory
- Movement and balance problems
- Learning difficulties (thinking, social skills, maths etc.)
- Speech and language delay
- Hearing and vision problems
- Problems with the liver, kidneys, heart and other organs
- Sleep and sucking problems as a baby
- Poor reasoning and judgement skills.

No general consensus on the 'low risk limit'

Scientists agree that heavy drinking is harmful. However, the 'safe limits' or 'low risk limits' recommended for alcohol intake vary remarkably across countries. One reason for this is the fact the knowledge in this area has evolved rapidly in the past two decades and is still evolving. While some countries have quickly embraced the new knowledge, others are yet to do so. It's likely that our knowledge in this area will continue to change significantly in the coming years.

My recommendation is that, if you don't drink, that is very good. Do not start to drink because you have read an article which outlines lots of benefits from drinking. While past studies have shown health benefits (reducing the risk of heart disease), recent studies show that this may have been exaggerated.[40] Furthermore, there is a risk that you can move from zero to heavy drinking, which would be terribly harmful. If you must drink, the key word is 'moderation'. You must moderate your alcohol intake to reduce your risks. Moderate alcohol use is defined differently in different countries, based on what is considered to be the 'low-risk limit'.

As an illustration of the variations in 'low risk limits', let's look at the UK and US guidelines for alcohol.

UK 'low risk limit' for alcohol

The UK guidance on alcohol (www.drinkaware.co.uk) recommends not drinking more than 14 units per week. Fourteen units are equivalent to a bottle and a half of wine or five pints of 5% beer. In the UK, alcohol intake is measured in units and one unit has 8 g of alcohol. A pint of 5.2% beer has 3 units, a pint of 3.6% beer has 2 units; a standard glass (175 ml) of 12% wine has 2 units and a large glass (250 ml) of 12% wine has 3 units. A large (35 ml) single measure of spirits has 1.4 units.

It's advisable that you limit the amount of alcohol you drink on any one occasion as binge drinking can, as we have seen, lead to injury, the misjudgement of risky situations and losing self-control. If you must have more than one drink, it's recommended that you drink more slowly, drink with food and alternate alcoholic drinks with water.

US 'low risk limit' for alcohol

The US Dietary Guidelines for Alcohol recommend a maximum of one drink per day for women and two drinks per day for men. A drink is equivalent to 5 ounces (147.8 ml) of 12% wine, 12 ounces (354.8 ml) of 5% beer, 8 ounces (236.6 ml) of 7% malt liquor, or 1.5 ounces (44.3 ml) of 80-proof distilled spirits or liquor.

People who should not drink at all

1. Women who are pregnant or may be pregnant.
2. People younger than 18 in the UK or 21 in the US. These are legal ages for alcohol consumption. However, it's important to note that the brain is not fully mature until age 25. Discouraging underage alcohol use is important to minimise alcohol-related disruption of brain development and decision-making capacity as well as to reduce negative behavioural consequences of alcohol consumption before neurobiological adulthood (25 years).[42]
3. People who have certain health conditions such as liver or heart disease or are taking certain medications such as antipsychotics or antibiotics that interact with alcohol.
4. Recovering alcoholics or people unable to control the amount they drink.
5. People who are doing things that require coordination, balance and alertness, such as driving or operating machinery.

Chapter Ten

Smoking

My childhood friend who is a physician told me he started smoking when he failed to get into medical school. When he eventually made it, he was already a smoker.

> **Lesson 10**
>
> Healthy and unhealthy habits formed when growing up are likely to continue later in life.

I asked my childhood friend who is a physician why he smoked. He told me that he had started when he was 18. He had been in his first year at the university having failed to get admission to medical school. He had enrolled on a course he didn't like. During that year, he had little interest in his studies. His dream of becoming a doctor seemed absurd. He started smoking. He had many friends who smoked like him. He smoked while we were together, but I never felt pressured to smoke.

One day he brought cigarettes with him. He lit one, sucked it for a few long seconds and sent the smoke vibrating out through his nostrils. It looked amazing and fun. 'You can try it,' he said, handing it over to me. I rejected the offer. That was the closest I ever came to smoking.

After one year of smoking and frustration, he got into the medical school, but by that time, he couldn't stop smoking easily. Smoking had become a habit. He continued to smoke throughout medical school and even as a physician. My experience taught me one big lesson. Healthy and unhealthy habits we form during teenage years and as young adults are likely to continue later in life.

There are many things to talk about with regard to smoking. I summarise the discussion that follows into three key points:
1. Smoking increases the risk of sick fat disease
2. Smoking takes a major toll on your health
3. Never smoke, but if you've started, quit.

Smoking increases the risk of sick fat disease

Active smoking increases the risk of developing sick fat disease (obesity, high blood pressure, high cholesterol and type 2 diabetes). Sick fat disease increases the risk of heart disease, stroke and blood clot formation. The risk of sick fat disease is increased by about 34% among active smokers. This risk is dose-dependent, meaning that it increases with the number of cigarettes smoked per day. The good thing is that cessation reduces the risk of sick fat disease. This means that if you stop smoking, your chances of developing sick fat disease will drop.

Smoking affects the four main components of sick fat disease:
1. obesity
2. blood pressure/cardiovascular system
3. cholesterol
4. diabetes.

1. Smoking and obesity

Smoking increases the risk of upper body or abdominal obesity. It is believed that chemicals in tobacco, such as nicotine, affect body-fat distribution, favouring the location of fat storage in the abdominal organs, such as the bowel, liver and kidneys. Smokers have been shown to have higher fasting blood levels of cortisol than non-smokers. High cortisol can lead to abdominal body fat storage. Female smokers show no absolute change in blood oestrogen concentrations but have higher levels of androgens (male hormones). In women, decreased oestrogen levels and increased testosterone levels, as seen during menopause, are associated with abdominal obesity. Conversely, smoking may decrease blood testosterone levels in men, a factor which is associated with abdominal obesity. Therefore, an imbalance between male and female sex hormones in women and a decrease in testosterone in men could play an important part in abdominal fat location observed in smokers.[43]

The ratio of waist to hip circumference, or WHR, is a good measure of upper body obesity. The normal value is less than 0.95 for men and 0.8 for women. Smokers and tobacco users tend to have a higher WHR than non-smokers.

2. Smoking and blood pressure/cardiovascular system

It's well established that smoking causes an acute increase in blood pressure (BP) and heart rate. However, the effect of chronic smoking on BP varies widely depending on the duration of exposure to cigarette smoke and the extent of the damage to blood vessels caused by nicotine and other chemicals in cigarette smoke.[44]

Smoking causes an acute increase in blood pressure and heart rate

The mechanism by which smoking affects blood pressure is still not fully understood but we know the effects are associated with both nicotine and carbon monoxide in cigarette smoke. The effects of the other more than 7000 chemicals isolated from cigarette smoke are still poorly understood.[45]

Studies suggest that there are several pathways by which smoking affects BP. Immediately after smoking, nicotine causes an increased heart rate, enhanced heart contractility and systemic vasoconstriction (narrowing of blood vessels thoughout the body), which all contribute to an immediate rise in BP. Nicotine has a direct vasoconstrictive effect on blood vessels and an indirect effect by causing the release of circulating catecholamines (adrenaline and noradrenaline) by the adrenal glands; these cause vasoconstriction and an increase in heart rate.[46]

After this acute phase following smoking, the BP may drop as a result of the depressant effects of chronic nicotine use. Nicotine causes the release of a hormone called beta-endorphin (a hormone that inhibits pain) by the pituitary gland in the brain. Beta-endorphin is an opioid hormone that induces euphoria. This euphoria is later replaced by a feeling of depression, low mood and fatigue, which forces the smoker to seek more nicotine. This cycle leads to chronic tobacco use and addiction. In addition to the depressant effects of nicotine, in the long term, the hypertensive action of nicotine may be offset by the hypotensive action of carbon monoxide. This explains why some studies have shown that people who smoke have a lower BP than non-smokers.[47]

Later, chronic cigarette smoking may damage blood vessels and increase artery stiffness, which may in turn cause the BP to increase again. Smoking increases the production of oxygen free radicals (such as superoxide anion radical) that damage blood vessels and decreases production of nitric oxide (a chemical that relaxes blood vessels causing them to widen). In response to smoke exposure, cells of the inner walls of blood vessels (endothelium) release inflammatory and 'proatherogenic' (atherosclerosis causing) cytokines which, together with free radicals, damage the endothelium. The damage to the endothelium is considered to be a key initiating event in the development of atherosclerosis (build-up of plaque consisting of fats, cholesterol and other substances in and on artery walls). Atherosclerosis can lead to heart disease and hardened arteries can in turn contribute to high blood pressure.[44]

Cigarette smoke contains extremely high levels of carbon monoxide. Research suggests that this odourless gas may affect the heart and blood vessels in two ways: first by oxygen deprivation and second by direct damage to heart and blood vessels, causing atherosclerosis. Carbon monoxide binds to haemoglobin, the molecule in red blood cells that carries oxygen from the lungs to tissues all over the body. When carbon monoxide binds to haemoglobin,, it forms carboxyhaemoglobin and oxygen can no longer bind. This decreases the amount of oxygen delivered to all cells and tissues. If tissues are deprived of oxygen (a situation called hypoxia), transient or permanent damage can occur, especially in those organs that demand high oxygen delivery, such as the brain and heart. In order to continue to deliver sufficient oxygen to tissues, the heart responds by increasing the rate at which it beats and its contractility, which in the long run may cause the heart to enlarge (cardiomegaly). Cardiomegaly increases the risk of sudden heart attack and heart failure. Animal studies suggest that carbon monoxide in cigarette smoke may act directly on the arterial wall and heart muscles causing oxidative stress and long-term irreversible structural damage.[48]

Active smokers usually have blood pressure which varies widely depending on the level of exposure to smoke and its effect on blood vessels. Many other factors related to lifestyle and genetic predisposition play a significant part in determining the level of BP. Passive smoking exposes individuals to the main smoking compounds, primarily nicotine, but also to carbon monoxide and other chemicals found in cigarette smoke. Passive, or secondhand, smokers inhale the same harmful chemicals as smokers. Therefore, passive smokers may experience the same detrimental effects on their cardiovascular system as smokers. Research evidence suggests that the rate of atherosclerotic change may be reduced by the cessation of smoking, but a residual effect appears to be present for a decade.[44]

3. Smoking and cholesterol

Cigarette smoking is associated with higher total cholesterol and triglyceride levels and lower levels of cardio-protective HDL cholesterol. The is a profile associated with atherogenesis (the formation of plaques in blood vessels), as we have seen. The mechanisms by which smoking affects blood fats are still incompletely understood, but several have been proposed.[49]

Nicotine and other poisons in tobacco increase LDL cholesterol and lower HDL cholesterol

First, smoking increases catecholamine (adrenaline and noradrenaline) release, causing a surge in circulating free fatty acids, which may increase LDL cholesterol and reduce HDL cholesterol.

Second, smoking reduces cholesterol acyl-transferase, the enzyme responsible for 'esterifying' free cholesterol and increasing the size of HDL particles. Cholesterol in the blood exists in two forms: free cholesterol and cholesteryl esters. Both of these are constituents of circulating LDL and HDL. High levels of free cholesterol may kill cells in part by inhibiting one or more cell membrane proteins whose function is either blocked or altered. Esterification of free cholesterol is one mechanism that removes it from cells and prevents its toxic effect.[50]

Third, another mechanism by which smoking affects cholesterol is by inhibiting 'reverse cholesterol transport', a mechanism that removes excess cholesterol from peripheral tissues and delivers it to the liver where it is removed from the body or redistributed to other tissues.[51]

Studies have consistently shown that smoking contributes to a poor cholesterol profile, with higher levels of LDL, lower levels of HDL and high triglycerides. Smoking cessation improves HDL cholesterol, total HDL and large HDL particles. Increases in HDL may partly be responsible for the reduced heart disease risk observed after quitting smoking.[49]

Smoking triggers an immunologic response to vascular injury, which is associated with increased levels of inflammatory markers, such as C-reactive protein, white blood cells and fibrinogen. Markers such as C-reactive protein are also increasingly implicated in the development (pathogenesis) of atherosclerosis and can predict heart disease.[52]

Smoking also increases the risk of blood clot formation (thrombosis) by increasing the synthesis of clotting factors, such as fibrinogen. Abstention from smoking for a period of only two weeks has been shown to induce a significant decrease in fibrinogen synthesis by the liver, with a matching reduction in blood concentrations of fibrinogen.[53]

4. Smoking and diabetes

Smoking and other tobacco uses (such as vaping) increase insulin resistance, the condition described earlier where insulin fails to mediate the uptake of sugar by the body's cells. This leads to type 2 diabetes. Even short-term tobacco use can lead to insulin resistance.[54] Smoking increases the risk of developing type 2 diabetes by 30 to 40%.[55] Managing diabetes and regulating insulin among smokers is more difficult because nicotine can lessen the effectiveness of insulin, causing smokers to need more insulin to regulate blood sugar levels.

Smoking reduces insulin sensitivity (which leads to insulin resistance) and impairs the functioning of pancreatic β-cells (the cells that produce insulin, as we have seen). While the mechanisms by which smoking contributes to diabetes are not fully understood, it's clear that nicotine and other chemicals in cigarette smoke induce inflammation and oxidative stress which can impact both on insulin sensitivity and β-cell function.

Furthermore, smoking also induces a stress response characterised by increased circulating levels of cortisol (the steroid hormone that increases blood glucose levels), increased release of catecholamines (adrenaline and noradremanlis, which cause an immediate increase in blood glucose), and increased growth hormone concentration (which decreases glucose oxidation and suppresses muscle uptake of glucose for short-term storage).[54]

How smoking takes a major toll on your health

In addition to contributing to sick fat disease, smoking and other tobacco uses are harmful to the body in many other ways. The effects can be summarised as:
- Smoking causes brain/neurological complications
- Smoking causes cancer
- Smoking causes lung disease
- Smoking causes pregnancy problems.

Though you may well be familiar with these issues, I believe it is important to state these risks here as part of the support for lifestyle change that I am advocating. Smoking increases the risk of several cancers including those of the lung, (and, less well known) oeosophagus, larynx, mouth, throat, kidneys, bladder, liver, pancreas, stomach, cervix, colon and rectum, and also of acute myeloid leukaemia. Moreover, toxic chemicals in cigarette smoke increase the risk of developing chronic obstructive pulmonary disease (COPD – chronic bronchitis and emphysema).

Smoking in pregnancy is known to increase the risk of congenital malformations, miscarriage, stillbirth, preterm birth, low birthweight and newborn death.

Finally, toxins from smoking increase the risk of developing neurological diseases such as multiple sclerosis, Alzheimer's disease, stroke and vascular dementia.

1. Smoking causes cancer

Cancer occurs when cells in our body grow rapidly out of control, creating a growth called a tumour. Poisons in cigarettes weaken the body's immune system. A weaker immune system means that the body cannot kill cancer cells, and so the cancer cells keep growing. Moreover, tobacco can damage or change the cells' DNA, which controls cell growth.

Nine out of 10 cases of lung cancer are caused by cigarette smoking. Smoking is also known to increase the risk of many other cancers. A large study of 422,010 participants followed for up to 30 years revealed that smoking increased the risk of several cancers, including lung cancer, liver cancer, bladder cancer, kidney cancer, pancreatic cancer, and lymphoma.[56]

Cigarette smoke contains a mixture of thousands of compounds, including more than 60 well-established carcinogens (cancer-causing chemicals). Carcinogens can cause DNA damage and gene mutations, which in turn can cause the loss of normal control of cell growth, ultimately resulting in excessive cell proliferation and cancer. Stopping smoking remains the only proven strategy for reducing the risk of smoking-induced cancers.[57]

2. Smoking causes lung disease

Smoking/tobacco use (e.g. vaping) and/or secondhand ('passive') smoking can cause a chronic lung condition called chronic obstructive pulmonary disease, or COPD. COPD is the term for a cluster of health conditions that cause airway blockage and breathing-related problems, including emphysema, asthma and chronic bronchitis. The toxins in cigarette smoke weaken your lungs' defence mechanisms against infections, cause swelling (inflammation) in the air passages and destroy air sacs (alveoli) where gases are exchanged in the lungs; these are all contributing factors for COPD.[58]

COPD reduces airflow through the airways, the tubes that carry air in and out of the lungs. The airways become inflamed and swollen and mucus can clog them. The airways are progressively destroyed. People with COPD may have symptoms such as cough, shortness of breath, tightness in the chest and wheezing.

Smoking during the teenage years can slow the development of the lungs and increase the risk of developing COPD in adulthood. In the US, eight out of 10 COPD-related deaths are caused by smoking.

3. Smoking causes pregnancy problems

Smoking and passive smoking can reduce the chances of getting pregnant and can cause infertility. They can damage the tissues of the unborn child and cause congenital malformations. Smoking can also cause miscarriage and preterm delivery. Babies whose mothers smoke can have low birth weight, and are at greater risk of 'cot death' (unexplained death during deep sleep). Smoking in pregnancy increases the risk of miscarriage, stillbirth, placental abruption (premature detachment of the placenta from the womb wall before delivery), preterm birth, low birthweight and neonatal morbidity (disease) and mortality (death). These adverse effects are primarily driven by carbon monoxide, tar and nicotine.[59]

Carbon monoxide from cigarette smoke rapidly binds to haemoglobin, forming carboxyhaemoglobin, This impairs oxygen delivery to the myometrium (muscles of the womb) and foetus.[59]

Tar is the combusted particulate substance contained in cigarette smoke which forms a residue on the lining of airways (mucous membranes) and lungs of smokers. Tar damages the airways by mechanical and biochemical mechanisms. It contains carcinogens which interfere with biochemical pathways inducing inflammation and with widespread oxidative damage. Animals studies show that tar is both foetotoxic (toxic to foetus) and teratogenic (causing congenital malformation). The Cadmium which is a heavy metal contained in cigarette smoke is known to accumulate in the placenta and to cause foetal growth restriction.[59]

Smoking or secondhand smoke can damage the tissues of the unborn child and cause congenital malformations

In addition to the effect on mother, nicotine readily crosses the placenta and has a direct effect on the foetus. Nicotine is a neuroteratogen (causing damage to brain and nervous system) and is known to alter normal brain development. It causes developmental damage including cognitive, emotional and behavioural problems in children of smokers, such as attention-deficit hyperactivity disorder and learning disabilities.[59]

4. Smoking causes brain/neurological complications

Smoking increases the risk of developing neurological complications, such as multiple sclerosis (in which the protective covering of nerve fibres is damaged by one's own immune system), Alzheimer's disease (progressive degeneration of brain cells impairing memory and other mental functions), stroke (a medical emergency which occurs when the blood supply to part(s) of the brain is interrupted or reduced) and vascular dementia (brain damage caused by multiple strokes leading to memory loss in older adults). Neurological damage caused by smoking is thought to be mediated by oxidative stress and inflammatory damage to both brain cells and blood vessels.

Normally, the blood–brain barrier prevents the passage of circulating toxins or pathogens from the blood to the brain, while at the same time allowing vital nutrients to reach the brain. The blood–brain barrier is the highly selective semi-permeable border of vascular endothelial cells (cells of the inner walls of blood vessels) that protect the brain. Nicotine is a toxic substance which, because of its lipid (fat) solubility, can cross the blood–brain barrier. Fat-soluble substances (including alcohol and caffeine, as well as nicotine) can dissolve in the cell membrane and cross the barrier, while substances that are soluble in water and not fat (such as penicillin) cannot. Nicotine causes cerebral vasodilation (expansion of blood vessels in the brain) and increased vascular permeability at the blood–brain barrier, facilitating the passage of unwanted substances, such as toxins and pathogens, from the blood into the brain. Chronic exposure to cigarette toxins induces oxidative stress, which can cause oxidative damage. Chronic smoking can trigger a strongly inflammatory cascade that can initiate the onset or facilitate the progression of neurological diseases.[60]

Never smoke, or quit smoking

Millions of people die each year from smoking. There are two proven ways to protect yourself and others:
- Never smoke
- Quit smoking!

Never smoke

It is better never to smoke than to try to quit smoking. Therefore, efforts should be made to prevent people from initiating smoking in the first place. Understanding the dangers of smoking, choosing friends who are non-smokers, managing your stress correctly, avoiding places where people smoke regularly and making a strong resolution never to start smoking, can all go a long way to prevent starting smoking.

Stress, anxiety and depression can cause people to start smoking. Once they start, they will continue after the initial problem is over. Like alcohol, smoking can be a negative coping mechanism for stress. It's strongly advisable not to indulge in smoking when one is stressed or is going through hard times.

Quit smoking

There are many benefits to giving up smoking. First, all the health risks and problems associated with smoking will be reversed and you will be healed. The sooner you quit, the better. Second, secondhand smoke harms others and one of the best things to do for your family is to quit smoking.

There are five reinforcing powers or accelerators for lasting smoking cessation (Ambition, Achievability, Amusement, Assistance and Approval):

- **Ambition:** You need to think positive and have faith and even passion that you will succeed. It doesn't matter if you have failed in the past. Make a list of reasons to quit smoking and develop a plan to quit.
- **Achievability:** You should be realistic about yourself and set goals that are achievable. Start small and think long-term, don't think big. For example, you can start be deciding to halve the number of cigarettes smoked per day if you think that is achievable. If you cannot quit smoking by yourself, seek help from a local 'stop smoking' service if available or from your doctor who can offer you nicotine replacement therapy.
- **Amusement:** Like every lifestyle change, you can make smoking cessation fun. Go out for a five-minute walk when you have a craving to smoke – go with a friend to make the walk more enjoyable. The various forms of

nicotine and e-cigarettes are all available and really can help you to quit smoking. Nicotine withdrawal can cause unpleasant symptoms when you try to quit smoking. Nicotine replacement therapy gives you the drug (in the form of gum, patches, sprays, inhalers, or lozenges) but not the other harmful chemicals in tobacco. Similar to nicotine replacement therapy are electronic cigarettes (e-cigarettes) which simulate tobacco smoking by vapourising tobacco. These generally contain fewer toxic chemicals than the deadly mix of more than 7000 chemicals found in smoke from regular cigarettes. Like nicotine replacement therapy, e-cigarettes are less harmful than regular cigarettes, but they are *not* safe. The main purpose is to help quit smoking.

- **Assistance:** You should inform your family members and friends about your plan to stop smoking. Acceptance by and assistance from friends and family members can help you. Join friends who want to stop smoking and build friendships with non-smokers. Local 'stop smoking' services can be of great help. Your doctor can prescribe nicotine replacement therapy, if you need it. Nicotine replacement therapy is available in the form of patches, gums, tablets, lozenges, nasal spray etc. Electronic cigarettes are also available where you use an electronic device that simulates tobacco smoking. With e-cigarettes, instead of smoke, you inhale vapour released by the device.
- **Approval:** You will need praise and recognition from others, whether it's your family members, friends or strangers. A single word of approval such as 'well-done' can make a big difference to your journey of smoking cessation.

Chapter Eleven

Stress

I made 10 long journeys in a year. When I looked back I noted that all the trips were stressful. No single journey was free of stress.

> **Lesson 11**
>
> Stressful events cannot be avoided since they occur without your wish, will or plan – but you have control over how you react to them.

After careful monitoring, I noticed that my BP was affected by two things: activity and stress. Mental activity, especially intense and prolonged mental work, caused my BP to rise. On the other hand, physical activity, such as gardening or cooking, caused my BP to drop.

Stress caused my BP to rise immediately. The increase in BP due to stress was much more on the systolic BP (upper value) than the diastolic BP (lower value). My BP rose when I was preparing for a major event, when I received a disturbing email, when I was involved in an argument, and with almost any nuisance. In fact, almost any daily hassle could cause my systolic BP to rise by about 5 to 10 mm Hg for a short time before dropping back to the non-stressed value.

I wasn't worried about small stressors because I found that some stress was actually good for me as it pushed me to do more than I would otherwise have done. However, I was worried about major stressful events and chronic stress as these do not only drain all your energy, but also are extremely harmful to the body. I asked myself the question: 'Is it possible to create a world free of stress?' If we could have a stress-free world, people would be far healthier than they are today.

In order to understand my daily stress better, I looked at my international flights in one year. I observed that I had taken 10 international trips in the previous year, involving 26 flights. In each of these trips, I had encountered multiple hassles which probably caused my BP to rise. In the 10 trips, six flights had been delayed, I had missed three, my luggage had been damaged in two, I had lost my luggage in one, there had been an emergency landing in one. Then my bank cards had failed to work on one trip, my hotel room had had multiple problems in three and there had been many more issues.

I learnt from my trips that we cannot avoid stress. We have to learn to live with it. We have to learn to manage stress. The world is filled with stress and in so far as we live in the present world, we will be stressed.

Murphy's Law:
Anything that can go wrong will go wrong

In fact, I now get suspicious if I am doing something and it is going smoothly without any nuisance or inconvenience that can cause stress. I manage my stress by managing my expectation. I set up my expectation that something is going to go wrong and very often it does. When it does, I am less stressed because I have been prepared for the worst. Indeed, to manage stress, Murphy's

Chapter Eleven

Law is useful: it states that 'anything that can go wrong will go wrong'.

Stress affects our health both directly and indirectly. I sum up the discussion that follows into three major points:
- Stress contributes to sick fat disease
- Stress takes a major toll on our health
- Stress management techniques can help.

Stress contributes to sick fat disease

Stress is a discomfort caused by any event or thought that makes us feel frustrated, angry or nervous – that we cannot cope. It is the body's way of reacting to a challenge or demand. The challenge or demand that causes the stress is called a stressor. Anxiety is stress that continues after the stressor is gone.

The body's reaction to stressors can be emotional, physical and/or behavioural.

Emotional symptoms of stress include feeling worried or anxious, low self-esteem, being irritable and moody, having racing thoughts and difficulty concentrating, depression, anxiety.

Physical symptoms include low energy, headaches, stomach upset, inability to sleep, low sex drive, dry mouth, muscle pains and weight gain or loss.

Behavioural symptoms include eating too much or too little, procrastinating and avoiding responsibilities, and increased use of alcohol, cigarettes or drugs.

The body's reaction to stressors can be emotional, physical and/or behavioural

Stress can contribute to sick fat disease either directly or indirectly. Indirectly, it does this by making people adopt unhealthy habits and directly, by activating two systems: the sympathetic nervous system (SNS) and the pituitary–adrenal axis (PAA).

The activation of these systems by stress triggers a chain of events that causes sick fat disease (abdominal obesity, high blood pressure, high cholesterol and type 2 diabetes). Common environmental stressors include unemployment, financial hardship, problems at work, family problems and social problems.

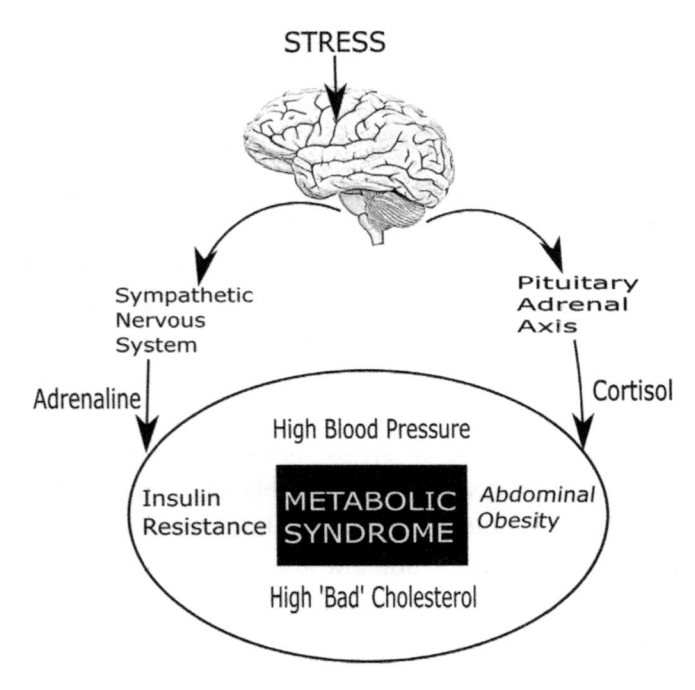

Figure 16: How stress causes sick fat disease directly

1. Sympathetic nervous system

Stress activates the sympathetic nervous system (SNS), the part of the body's nervous (electrical) system responsible for the 'fight or flight' response. The SNS causes the release of adrenaline which increases the heart rate, breathing, blood flow to the muscles, sweating and blood pressure. Chronic stress leads to sustained activation of the SNS which causes sustained high blood pressure.

2. Pituitary–adrenal axis

Stress activates the pituitary–adrenal axis (also called hypothalamic–pituitary–adrenal axis) which leads to the release of cortisol from the adrenal glands. The normal stress response starts within seconds and might last for days before everything is back to normal. However, with chronic stress the release of cortisol is prolonged and this leads to abdominal obesity, type 2 diabetes and high cholesterol levels.

How stress takes a major toll on your health

Stress can be acute or chronic. Acute stress is short-lived and goes away very quickly. It's necessary to keep you motivated and to enable you to meet deadlines. It occurs every time and is actually useful.

Chronic stress lasts for a longer period of time, often weeks or months. It's often caused by a chronic stressor such as trouble at work or an unhappy marriage. Chronic stress may lead to serious health problems.

Post-traumatic stress disorder (PTSD) is a health condition due to failure to recover after experiencing or witnessing a terrifying event. It may last for months or years with triggers that bring back memories of the trauma. Symptoms of PTSD include nightmares, flashbacks, anxiety, depression, mood swings and avoidance of those triggers.

Post-traumatic stress disorder (PTSD) is a health condition due to failure to recover after experiencing or witnessing a terrifying event

When stress is short-lived, it enables the body to deal with environmental threats or challenges. However, when stress becomes chronic, it is harmful to the body. Chronic stress contributes to sick fat disease by activating the sympathetic nervous system and the pituitary–adrenal axis, as described on page 147. It affects our brain (nervous system), defence (immune) system, endocrine (hormonal) system and digestive (gut) system. In summary, its negative effects are:

- Digestive (modifies appetite, bowel movements and absorption; increases inflammation)
- Immune (weakens the immune system)
- Nervous (kills brain cells and causes the brain to shrink)
- Endocrine (activates adrenaline and cortisol release, and suppresses the release of growth hormone)
- Sick fat disease (activates sympathetic nervous system and cortisol release).

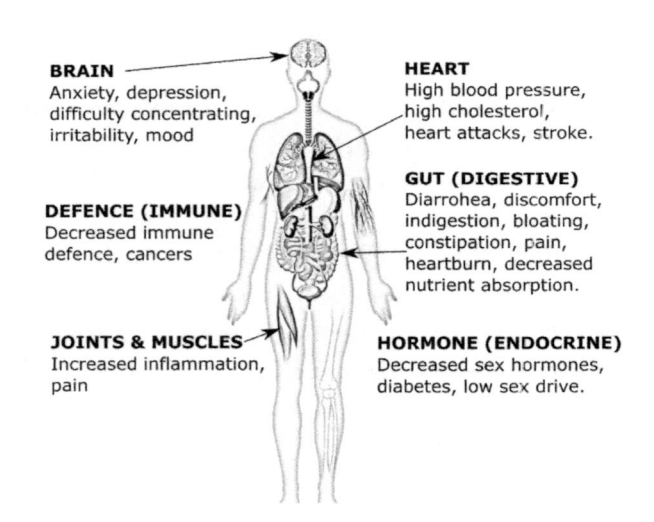

BRAIN
Anxiety, depression, difficulty concentrating, irritability, mood

HEART
High blood pressure, high cholesterol, heart attacks, stroke.

DEFENCE (IMMUNE)
Decreased immune defence, cancers

GUT (DIGESTIVE)
Diarrohea, discomfort, indigestion, bloating, constipation, pain, heartburn, decreased nutrient absorption.

JOINTS & MUSCLES
Increased inflammation, pain

HORMONE (ENDOCRINE)
Decreased sex hormones, diabetes, low sex drive.

Figure 17: The effects of stress on the body

Chapter Eleven

1. Stress and the digestive system

Chronic stress adversely affects the digestive system in four ways: by modifying appetite, by modifying bowel movements, by modifying absorption and by increasing inflammation.

Stress can either increase or reduce appetite. Increase in appetite can lead to obesity; reduction in appetite can lead to the person becoming underweight. Stress modifies bowel movements and this can lead to constipation and bloating. It also increases stomach acid secretion and reduces water absorption, which can cause diarrhoea. It increases inflammation generally and can therefore cause or aggravate inflammation of the bowel.

2. Stress and the immune system

Chronic stress weakens the body's immunity and makes us more vulnerable to illness. This is because the stress hormone cortisol suppresses the immune system. The risk of disease appearing soon after a sudden, major and extremely stressful life event, such as divorce or the loss of a job, is very high.

By suppressing our immunity, chronic stress can cause cancer. Our immune system normally produces specialised cells (such as natural killer (NK) cells) that destroy cancer cells and prevent the spread of cancer in its early stages. Stress reduces the activity of NK and other immune cells and allows cancer to develop and spread.

> *By suppressing our immunity, chronic stress can cause cancer*

Chronic stress also promotes what we call autoimmunity (literally 'self' immunity), where the immune system attacks the body's own tissues. Imagine a war where the army fires on its own troops by mistake causing self-inflicted casualties ('friendly fire'). This is exactly what happens during autoimmunity. Stress makes the immune system believe that the body's tissues are foreign bodies ('antigens'), just like viruses and bacteria.[61] The immune system therefore sends its soldiers called antibodies to attack the body's tissues. This leads to autoimmune diseases such as rheumatoid arthritis (joint inflammation).

How stress contributes to autoimmunity is not fully understood. One explanation is that chronic stress simultaneously enhances and suppresses different aspects of the immune response by altering patterns of cytokine secretion, as follows. Stress activates the sympathetic nervous system (see page 151). Some sympathetic nerve fibres descend from the brain into the thymus gland, which secretes cytokines. Cytokines secreted by Th1 cells in the thymus (such as interleukins 4, 5 and 13) are suppressed by stress. Th1 cytokines (suppressed by stress) normally activate cell immunity, which provides our defence against many kinds of infection and some kinds of cancer. On the other hand, chronic stress elicits the production of Th2 cytokines by the thymus, which activates antibody immunity and exacerbates allergy and many kinds of autoimmune disease.[61]

3. Stress and the nervous system

Stress causes brain tissue to die and waste away or break down. This is called brain atrophy. Atrophy affects our ability to learn and also causes emotional problems.
- Learning disorders: problems with memory, attention, decision-making, ability to concentrate, judgement, etc
- Emotional disorders: anxiety, depression, loss of self-confidence, mood swings etc.

Brain areas involved in the stress circuit (the hippocampus, amygdala, and pre-frontal cortex) undergo atrophy (wasting/shrinkage) with chronic stress. The hippocampus is principally responsible for long-term memory, but also mediates emotional responses. The amygdala is part of the brain that drives the 'fight or flight' response, but also plays a pivotal role in memory. The pre-frontal cortex contributes to a wide variety of functions including coordination, planning for the future, anticipating the consequences of one's action, personality expression, decision-making, moderating social behaviour, and moderating certain aspects of speech and language.

Stress-induced brain atrophy is believed to be caused by stresss-related changes, including elevated levels of cortisol, inhibition of neurogenesis (formation of new brain cells), increased levels of glutamate (normal amounts modulate brain functions like memory and learning, but excess glutamate causes over-excitation of brain cells and eventually cell death) and/or decreased levels of nerve growth factor (which is critical for brain cell multiplication/proliferation and survival).[62]

4. Stress and the endocrine system

The endocrine (or, as I call it, 'key worker') system produces hormones. Hormones (chemical messengers) are the 'key workers' that do the essential work without which we cannot stay alive. Stress affects the activity of our endocrine system. It causes the release of adrenaline and cortisol from the adrenal glands by activating the sympathetic nervous system and the pituitary–adrenal axis. It decreases insulin production by the pancreas, which may contribute to stress-induced hyperglycaemia (elevated blood sugar) and diabetes. By activating the sympathetic nervous system and the pituitary–adrenal axis which leads to increased cortisol secretion, stress inhibits thyroid-stimulating hormone (TSH) secretion and the production of thyroid hormones (T3 and T4), which can contribute to hypothyroidism (underactive thyroid). Acute stress increases levels of growth hormone by the pituitary gland. Growth hormone acts on tissues to increase metabolism and growth. However, prolonged psychosocial stress has the opposite effect on growth hormone. It suppresses its release by the pituitary gland which can lead to short stature in children. Stress can therefore have serious effects in children by inhabiting their development and growth. It also lowers sex hormones (testosterone and oestrogens) and this can cause infertility and disruption of the normal menstrual cycle.[63]

4. Stress and sick fat disease

Cortisol released in response to stress causes excess fat storage in the abdomen. This leads to abdominal, or apple-shaped, obesity which increases the risk of sick fat disease, as we have seen.

The mechanisms by which cortisol promotes the deposition of fat in the abdomen ('visceral fat storage') instead of the lower body (sub-cutaneous) is still not fully understood, but it is thought that abdominal fat depots are more responsive to cortisol due to their high glucocorticoid receptor expression (that is, receptors to which cortisol and other glucocorticoids bind) compared with subcutaneous fat. Cortisol increases the expression of numerous genes involved in fat deposition. There is growing scientific evidence that it has multiple, depot-dependent effects on fat cell gene expression and metabolism that promote abdominal fat deposition.[64]

The activation of the sympathetic nervous system by stress causes high blood pressure due to the sustained release of adrenaline causing an increase in heart rate and narrowing of the blood vessels.

Chronic stress has an indirect effect on cholesterol levels. It increases unhealthy dietary habits and obesity, both of which can cause an increase in LDL cholesterol.

Stress leads to sick fat disease, both directly and indirectly, by causing us to adopt unhealthy habits

Chronic stress causes a rise in blood sugar levels in several ways:
1. First, cortisol inhibits insulin secretion by the pancreas by acting on pancreatic α and β cells to modulate the secretion of glucagon and insulin, the two hormones that play a pivotal role in the regulation of blood glucose levels.[65]
2. Second, cortisol increases the synthesis of glucose by the liver (by inhibiting the activity of the enzyme glycogen synthase), which elevates circulating glucose concentrations.
3. Third, adrenaline released by activation of the sympathetic nervous system, promotes the breakdown of glycogen to sugar (glycogenolysis) in the muscles by activating the hormone, glycogen phosporylase.
4. Fourth, adrenaline inhibits the insulin-mediated conversion of blood sugar to glycogen in the muscles.
5. Fifth, cortisol stimulates fat breakdown (lipolysis) in fatty tissues to release fatty acids for energy production in tissues, such as the liver. This increases free fatty acids in the blood. Excess free fatty acids become incompletely metabolised because fat breakdown is activated up-stream but downstream processes in the metabolic chain are not activated. The accumulation of incompletely metabolised fats in cells (mitochondria) impairs insulin-signalling and leads to insulin resistance.[66] (As we have seen, when insulin is available in large amounts in the blood but can't do its job, we call this condition insulin resistance or insulin insensitivity. Eventually, blood sugar levels rise to abnormal levels, leading to full blown type 2 diabetes.)

Stress management techniques

Various techniques have been used successfully to manage stress. The best to use depends on the severity of the problem.

Moderate stress can be relieved by exercise, meditation, rest and relaxation, diet modification (such as decreasing the intake of alcohol and caffeine), support groups and social bonds with family and friends. Severe stress may require psychotherapy to uncover and address the root causes.

Emergency stress stoppers help you to control your reaction to an external pressure or stressor (trigger). I find the following very helpful in interrupting such triggers:

- I count from 1 to 10 before I speak or react.
- I take a few slow, deep breaths until I feel relaxed.
- I go out for a walk even if it's just for 5 minutes.
- I sleep on it and respond the next day, if it's not urgent.
- I pray. If you don't pray, you can meditate.
- I turn on some chill music or an inspirational podcast.

Using emergency stress stoppers doesn't guarantee that you will completely avoid stress. If you still experience its symptoms, there are some techniques that can help you manage it. Chronic stress is EMOTIONALLY damaging. Techniques to manage stress are EMOTIONALLY relieving.

E = Exercise
M = Music (play)
O = Occupy yourself
T = Take control
I = Improve your diet
O = Optimistic (be…)
N = Network
A = Accept
L = Labour smarter (not harder)
L = Lighten up
Y = Yoga (meditate/pray)

Chapter Eleven

These are the 11 EMOTIONALLY relieving stressbusters that can help you manage stress:

1. *Exercise:* Exercise is a well-known technique that I use every day to relieve me of light to moderate stress.
2. *Music (play):* I listen to music or watch an inspirational performance. If you play an instrument yourself that can be even better.
3. *Occupy yourself:* I challenge myself by setting up a goal to accomplish. I try to keep myself busy.
4. *Take control* of the situation. By remaining passive, the stress will just get worse. I try to take action and do something about the issue rather than remaining helpless. This is exactly what I did when I was diagnosed with diabetes and high blood pressure.
5. *Improve your diet:* I avoid unhealthy eating habits such as overeating, and drinking too much alcohol and caffeine when I am stressed. These will simply make things worse.
6. *Optimistic (be...):* I try to be positive; I focus on the positives and things I am grateful for. I write down a few things that went well for which I am grateful.
7. *Network:* I maintain a good network of family, colleagues and friends to provide a strong support that will relieve my stress. This social support system helps me to relax and feel that I am not alone. I also find that helping others helps to prevent or relieve my stress.
8. *Accept:* I accept the situation as it is if I don't have, and can't take, control. Everything has an end; it's just a matter of time.
9. *Labour smarter (not harder):* I don't try to do everything. Instead I prioritise my work and focus on things that are really important and will help me achieve my goal. This means working smarter, not harder.

10. *Lighten up:* I relax and do something that I really enjoy. I try to have some time of my own, say two nights per week, during which I forget about work and relax.
11. *Yoga (meditate/pray):* You can practise yoga, meditate or pray. For me, I pray and I find that prayers work very well against stress.

Chapter Twelve

Try, track and tell

I couldn't agree more with Steve Jobs when he said 'Stay hungry, stay foolish'. By staying hungry or curious for knowledge, and by believing that I wasn't an expert (staying foolish), I finally learned a lot about myself and my health.

> **Lesson 12**
>
> While your doctor is an expert on medicine, you are an expert on you; so stay hungry, stay foolish about your health.

I didn't want my doctor to do everything for me. I wanted to have more control over my own health. I was hungry for knowledge, both the knowledge that science has generated over centuries and the knowledge that I could create myself. In addition, I decided to be a fool and try out everything, without trusting that I was a doctor myself and assuming I knew the answers.

The first 30 trials I put myself through helped me to uncover the cure for type 2 diabetes. I continued with up to 70 trials to find a cure for high blood pressure. I didn't stop at 70. I continue to try out different things. I still follow my three simple steps of 'try, track and tell'. These are the 3Ts of trial and error.

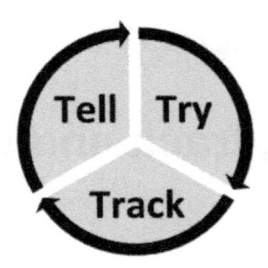

Figure 18: The 3Ts of trial and error

I 'try' different things, 'track' or monitor my BP, weight and workouts/physical activity, and 'tell' what works and what doesn't. Each person is different, so it is important that you 'track and tell' your personal response to whatever you do to confirm whether or not it works for you.

When you are exercising and trying to lose weight, it is important that you track your progress. You need to know your current level so that you can set a goal that you can gradually attain. Important measures you might consider tracking are:
- Steps, distance and calories
- Weight, BMI and waist-to-hip ratio (WHR)
- Blood pressure
- Annual health check.

Steps, distance and calories

Steps, distance and calories are measures used to track your workouts and physical activity.

Steps

Tracking how many steps you take per day can be a useful way to determine how active you are. A study showed that healthy people generally take between 4000 and 18,000 steps per day. An average of 10,000 is used by many people and is

also incorporated in many step-tracking apps though there is no published evidence to support this 'magic number'. Steps are easy to track because you can simply use your smart phone to record how many steps you are taking per day. Many smart phones come with health apps already installed, but you can also look for one from Google Play Store or App Store and install. You can also buy a speedometer to track steps, distance and calories burnt. As a simple guide, consider:
- Less than 5000 steps per day = inactive
- 5000 to 9999 steps per day = average
- 10,000 or more steps per day = very active.

Steps are easy for everybody because you don't need special shoes or exercise equipment and you don't have to count the steps by yourself. The challenge with steps is that they don't tell you the type of exercise you are doing. For example, if you have taken 10,000 steps while walking slowly, there will have been little impact on your heart. However, if the same 10,000 steps were attained while running, you will have a significant positive effect on your heart.

Nevertheless, counting steps is the starting point. You don't need to begin immediately with 10,000 steps. You can increase the steps progressively, by about 1000 per day every two weeks, until you reach your goal.

2. Distance

Another way to track your physical activity is to measure the distance you cover each day: 10,000 steps correspond to approximately 5 miles (8 km), so healthy people walk between 2 and 9 miles per day. In 2012 it was estimated that an average American walks 1.5 to 2 miles per day, which is approximately 3000 to 4000 steps.[67]

As with the steps you take, the distance you cover per day can be tracked using health apps on your smart phone. In fact, steps are converted to distance and to calories burnt. Like steps, the distance covered can't tell us much about the type of physical activity. If you have sick fat disease, you want to make sure that you are engaged in aerobic exercises of moderate to vigorous intensity. Low intensity exercises do not increase your heart rate and breathing and therefore are not considered to have 'cardio' effects, although they still have general health benefits, including some improvements in the heart.

3. Calories burnt

You can also track the calories you burn each day using the health apps on your smart phone or speedometer. Some exercise machines, such as treadmills, can also estimate calories burnt, distance covered and steps walked. The actual number of calories burnt per mile depends on the weight of the person and how fast the persons moves. There are free walking calorie calculators online that can do the calculations for you.

A rule of thumb is that 65 calories are burnt per mile by a 120-pound person and 100 calories are burnt per mile by a 180-pound person

Your weight is more important in calories burnt than your speed. A rule of thumb is that 65 calories are burnt per mile by a 120-pound (54.5 kg) person and 100 calories are burnt per mile by a 180-pound (81.6 kg) person.

Weight, BMI and waist-to-hip ratio (WHR)

To measure the actual impact of physical activity and diet on weight loss, you need to track your weight, BMI (body mass index) and/or WHR (waist-to-hip ratio).

Chapter Twelve

1. Weight

Your weight, of course, is the easiest way to track a weight-loss plan. It can vary during the day depending on many factors, including your food or water intake and activity levels. You need to get a good balance to be sure the measurements are accurate. You can measure your weight twice a day and take the average to give you a better idea of your weight. When you start a weight-losing exercise and diet plan, give yourself enough time for your body to burn your fat stores so that you can start seeing the impact on your weight.

Weight doesn't tell you the complete story. It doesn't tell you whether or not you are overweight or obese. It also doesn't tell you where your fat stores are located. As we have seen, fat located in the lower body (hips and thighs) is less unhealthy than fat located in the upper body (abdomen).

2. BMI

BMI, or body mass index, is calculated by dividing weight (in kilograms) by the square of the person's height (in metres). It is expressed in units of kg/m^2. It is a measure of body fat. It therefore has an advantage over weight in that it can tell whether a person is underweight, normal weight, overweight or obese.

$$\text{Body mass index} = \frac{\text{Weight (kg)}}{\text{Height} \times \text{Height (m}^2)}$$

Underweight = BMI less than 18.5
Normal weight = BMI 18.5 to 24.9
Overweight = BMI 25 to 29.9
Obese = BMI equal to or greater than 30

BMI has been used since the 1830s. It was first devised by Lambert Adolphe Jacques Quetelet, a Belgian mathematician, astronomer and sociologist, to determine whether a person had a healthy weight. However, BMI still doesn't tell the entire story. It doesn't tell us where excess body fat is located. Therefore, it doesn't reliably predict whether the person is at risk of falling ill. As described above, we know that lower body obesity is protective while upper body obesity increases the risk of sick fat disease.

3. *Waist-to-hip ratio*

Waist-to-hip ratio, or WHR, is defined as the waist circumference divided by the hip circumference. For example, if a person has a waist circumference of 80 cm and a hip circumference of 100 cm, then their WRH is 0.8. The WHR measures abdominal fat (upper body obesity) and therefore is more reliable than BMI in predicting ill health. Hip circumference or perimeter is measured around the lowest portion of the buttocks. Waist circumference is measured by placing the tape just above the hipbones (at the sides) and just below the navel/belly button (in front).

The WHR is a measure of the likelihood of a person developing a serious health condition, such as high blood pressure, type 2 diabetes and/or heart disease.

$$\text{Waist-to-hip ratio} = \frac{\text{Waist circumference}}{\text{Hip circumference}}$$

Normal WHR = less than 0.9 for men and less than 0.8 for women

Overweight WHR = 0.9 to 0.99 for men and 0.8 to 0.84 for women

Obese WHR = 1 or greater for men and 0.85 or greater for women.

Blood pressure

Blood pressure (BP) is a measure of the force with which the blood pushes against the walls of the blood vessels. As we have seen, it is measured by two values. The upper (higher) value, called systolic BP, measures the force with which the heart pumps blood into the blood vessels. The lower value, called diastolic BP, is a measure of the resistance to blood flow in the blood vessels. BP is considered normal when it's between 90/60 and 120/80 mm Hg (that is, millimetres of mercury as blood pressure meters used to use a column of mercury).

Normal BP is between 90/60 and 120/80 mm Hg

You are considered to have high BP if it is 140/90 mm Hg or higher. A BP of between 120/80 mm Hg and 140/90 mm Hg is considered elevated and could mean either you have chronically high BP or you are at risk of developing it.

In order to significantly reduce your BP, you need to undertake regular moderate to vigorous intensity exercise for several months. The lower BP associated with regular aerobic and strength-building exercises is thought to be driven largely by reduction in vascular (blood vessel) resistance. The endothelium (inner wall of blood vessels) in exercising muscles produces nitric oxide and prostacyclin, both of which promote enhanced vasodilatation by relaxing the smooth muscle cells in the blood vessel walls.[68] In addition, the structure of the heart adapts to regular aerobic exercise by increasing its mass, while maintaining or even enhancing its contractile (pumping) function.[68] When your heart is adequately trained to pump your blood, you can say 'goodbye' to antihypertensive medications. You need to track your BP because you may need to adjust the amount of exercise you take based on how your high BP responds to the exercise.

As mentioned in Chapter 7, I observed that sweat-inducing exercise lowers BP more than any exercise that doesn't cause sweating. Sweating induced by exercise causes the loss of water and salt, including sodium. The loss of sodium through sweat lowers BP.

Furthermore, ageing leads to progressive impairment of the functioning of the endothelium (inner walls of blood vessels) and reduction of nitric oxide production (which dilates blood vessels, lowering BP, as we have seen). People who exercise regularly show a slower decline in endothelial function and more gradual drop in nitric oxide than people who do not. This suggests that exercise helps keep arteries young.[69]

The mechanism by which exercise helps in keeping arteries young is still incompletely understood. Animal research shows that it stimulates the bone marrow (tissue inside our bones that produces blood cells) to produce endothelial progenitor cells, which enter the bloodstream to replace ageing endothelial cells and repair damaged arteries. People with coronary artery disease who have high levels of endothelial progenitor cells in their blood have been found to be protected from heart attacks and death from heart disease.[70]

Annual health check results

The frequency of health checks varies from country to country. I recommend that you go for an annual health check if you are over 40. A good health check takes approximately 30 minutes. It is conducted by a health professional – a doctor, nurse or healthcare assistant, depending on the country. Such a check is important for two reasons. First, it assesses your risk of developing serious health conditions such as high blood pressure, type 2 diabetes, kidney disease, stroke, heart disease and cancer. Second, it can pick up any of these conditions at an early stage.

A health check consists of three parts:
1. Questions
2. Clinical examination
3. Laboratory tests

Chapter Twelve

The health professional will ask you questions about your family history and lifestyle. This helps assess your risk of developing a serious health condition. Clinical examination includes checking your weight, blood pressure and general health condition. Finally, laboratory tests are conducted to screen for any health issues.

A health check can pick up serious health conditions and potentially prevent untimely death

In the UK, you can have your health check with your GP.

Chapter Thirteen

Changing your lifestyle

While it took me three months to lose 10 kilos, it took me over five years to move from a sedentary to a physically active lifestyle. I identified five key things that helped me to change.

> **Lesson 13**
>
> Five mutually reinforcing forces or motivators (the 5As – ambition, achievability, amusement, assistance and approval) are necessary to break old habits and form new ones.

I moved from zero exercise per day to one hour of moderate to vigorous intensity exercise. It took me five years to achieve this level of performance because I hated exercise. I hated all forms of manual work.

Unlike exercise, I personally found it easier to fast and to reduce my calorie intake than to exercise. As I've described, I lost 10 kg of weight in three months. My weight has since remained at 70 kg following the loss of 10 kg. It took me much longer to achieve a desirable performance in exercise. Now, come rain or shine, I do my exercises every day – I run and jog for at least one hour.

Because I struggled so hard to be able to do exercise, I learnt a lot in the process. Indeed, I sincerely believe there are few people, if any, who hate exercise as much as I did. That is why the first five years of my exercise struggle focused on normal walking, not even brisk walking. I had to start small, and build strength and confidence. So, what did I do to change from a sedentary to a very active lifestyle? My experience and lessons learnt can be summarised into five key points which I call the five As, or 'accelerators' (motivators) of behavioural change:

- Ambition
- Achievability
- Amusement
- Assistance
- Approval.

Ambition

My ambition or drive to do exercise was very strong. First, I believed that the long-term consequences of living with diabetes and high blood pressure were life-threatening. Second, I believed that exercise and weight loss would reduce the risks. Third, I believed that I could overcome the barriers to exercise. Although I hated exercise, I knew that exercising daily was far better than facing the consequences of diabetes and high blood pressure.

Behaviour change starts with motivation

Behaviour change starts with motivation. If you don't have the drive or motivation to change, forget about it. Motivation comes naturally if you are concerned about the threat, you believe that what you are going to do will work and you believe that you are capable of overcoming any barriers that could hinder you from changing. A strong motivation lays the foundation for a lasting change in lifestyle.

Chapter Thirteen

Achievability

All entrepreneurs are familiar with the concept 'start small, think big'. My experience with behaviour change is that you 'start small, think long term'. Achievability is about making sure you think more about sustaining the change, rather than moving quickly. When I started with exercise, if someone had told me that I needed to dream that one day I would be running one hour every day, I would have got discouraged and abandoned everything. Instead, I wasn't thinking big. I focused on thinking long term. Everything that I did, I made sure I was confident that I could do it for the rest of my life. I didn't want to start anything that I would slide back from after a few weeks or months. I found myself increasing my exercise goals, but that came naturally, not because I planned to raise the bar. I planned not to slide back.

With behaviour change, 'start small, think long term'

Before starting exercise, I was doing between 1000 and 2000 steps every day. My first target was to attain 4000 steps per day. At that time, I believed if I did the 4000 steps per day, I would be fine. I had no idea that I would one day go above this number. However, I knew that whether it rained or not, I had to do those 4000 steps.

After a few months of doing 4000 steps, I felt comfortable to move up to 5000. Over four years, I moved progressively from 4000 to 10,000 steps per day. I didn't increase the number of steps if I was not feeling confident that I would maintain that level of exercise.

I topped up the number of steps to 10,000 per day when I came back from work. When I anticipated challenges, I walked my 10,000 steps in the morning instead of evening. I could walk and complete the 10,000 steps in the living room, garden, park or anywhere. There was no reason for me not to complete my steps because to do so didn't need any special shoes, equipment or place.

Amusement

Exercise can be boring and repetitive, especially to those who hate it. It doesn't have to be. You can make your exercise fun. I initially made my exercise fun by counting the number of steps I took. When I had counted up to 100, I re-started from one. I noted how many hundreds I had made. This helped me know how close I was to my goal of 10,000. This kept me motivated as I approached my target.

Later on I added workout music. Now I run or jog to the rhythm of the music and this is really fun. I always use the same music (a motivational fitness song); it is exactly one hour, three minutes. From the music, I can detect when I have exercised for 20 minutes, 30 minutes, 40 minutes or 50 minutes. I also keep counting my steps, while the music is playing. The rhythmic synchronisation of the steps, counting and musical beats provides the momentum and energy that drive the exercise.

You can make your exercise fun

There are many other ways to make exercise fun. Some of the things you can try are exercising with friends, using a fitness tracker, expanding your list of exercises, using workout videos, exercising outdoors, rewarding yourself and using apps that make exercise amusing. Each person is different. What is fun to one person may not be to another. So, you need to try out several options and identify what works best for you.

Assistance

When you embark on a lifelong change, you need support from your family and friends. You need their acceptance and assistance. When I started exercising, I explained to my wife and kids what I would be doing and why. They knew that exercising was a healthy habit and were happy that I was determined to embark on such a lifestyle change. Positive words from them, such as 'good job', 'you're a star', 'well done', 'I wish I could be like you', 'you're very disciplined', kept me going. Their encouragement was particularly helpful when I was down and feeling like I shouldn't do any exercise. There are times when they join me on these routine exercises and this makes me stay motivated and committed. I find it fun exercising with them.

Support for physical activity from family and friends helps us exercise more and sustain fitness habits

One other person who supported me a lot was my sister-in-law, Charlotte. She made me work harder. She wanted to lose weight and embarked on an intensive exercise plan in which she did two to four hours of moderate to vigorous intensity exercise per day. She would do one to two hours in the morning and one to two hours in the evening. I felt challenged by the fact that I was only walking. I did my 10,000 steps only walking and the most I could do was brisk walking. For most of the time it was just normal walking. I joined her for her early-morning workouts in the park. We jogged and ran round the football field. The first week was very difficult. I felt pains in my joints, especially my knees and ankles. I sweated profusely. After two weeks, the pains in my joints disappeared. I had proved that I was capable. I gained more confidence. Since then I've never missed a day without doing my one hour of jogging and running.

Studies have shown that support for physical activity from family and friends helps people exercise more and sustain fitness habits. Exercising with others has many advantages including:
- It makes exercise more fun

- It makes you work harder
- It helps you build new friendships
- It helps you sustain your fitness habits
- Others may give you more exercise ideas
- It is safer to exercise with someone else
- It helps you to achieve your goals.

You may also need the assistance of a coach or counsellor to help you adopt the appropriate lifestyle. Seek assistance if necessary.

Approval

The power of approval, praise and recognition cannot be over-estimated. One month after changing from walking to jogging and running, I was in the park on my regular early morning run. I had run round the football field 15 times and was feeling really exhausted. There was a group of young men in their early 20s using the playground swings and messing about. As I approached, one of them quickly climbed over the fence of the playground and stood pretty much in my way. It looked like he was going to attack me and I felt nervous, but when I got about three meters away from him, he spoke to me: 'Congratulations, man! We admire you. None of us here can do what you've done! You've run round the pitch so many times – unbelievable!'

Praise is very powerful, especially when it is unexpected. It should be proportional to the effort

These words energised me. I felt like an Olympic star. In just one month, I was able to do physical activity that 'normal' people would find extraordinary. I gained confidence. That day

Chapter Thirteen

I ran round the field 30 times and went home feeling as if I were just starting the exercise. Over the next several months, my confidence grew. I recall occasions when I stayed in hotels and went to the gyms there. I would run on the treadmill for an hour or more. As easy as it seemed, I found that people were amazed by my level of endurance. Many who arrived at the gym after me would leave before me.

Praise is very powerful, especially when it is unexpected. It should be proportional to the effort, otherwise it loses its value.

Chapter Fourteen

A healthy living environment

I knew as a teenager that smoking, alcohol misuse, excessive calorie intake, unhealthy foods and physical inactivity were bad. The awareness didn't prevent me from developing sick fat disease.

> **Lesson 14**
>
> In order to adopt a healthy lifestyle, you need a favourable environment that empowers you to live such a lifestyle.

As a teenager, I learnt a lot about living healthily. I knew I had to eat healthy foods, avoid smoking, moderate my alcohol intake, take exercise and manage stress. As a medical student, these things were reinforced and taught about in different courses. However, this knowledge fell on deaf ears. Knowledge alone does not bring about the adoption of a healthy lifestyle. The environment is too powerful and very often ignored.

Lifestyle is affected by the home where a child grows, the community where he/she lives, schools attended, what is fashionable at the time, just to mention a few factors. These are powerful but sometimes invisible forces that affect aspects of lifestyle, whether exercise, healthy eating, smoking or alcohol intake.

Knowledge alone cannot bring about the adoption of a healthy lifestyle. The environment is too powerful and very often ignored

While I knew that being overweight could increase my risk of sick fat disease, in my community most adults were either overweight or obese. Over time, my subconscious mind accepted that being overweight was 'normal' and that perhaps it was the science that was wrong to classify everyone as overweight or obese. With this embedded in my subconscious mind, I saw my being overweight as 'normal', until I developed sick fat disease. When I lost 10 kg and reversed my diabetes, that was when I was convinced that being overweight was not normal and could cause sick fat disease.

Governments have a critical role in shaping the environment in which we live in order to prevent sick fat disease. This disease is responsible for millions of deaths globally each year. A quarter of these deaths are premature, occurring between the ages of 30 and 70. Low- and middle-income countries account for almost 90% of these premature deaths. The resulting economic losses amount to trillions of US dollars and millions of people are trapped in poverty.

The environment is the habitat in which we live. Our HABITAT has a major role in determining whether or not we get sick fat disease.

Environment means HABITAT
- **H** = **H**ome
- **A** = **A**rea (where we live)
- **B** = **B**usinesses (around us)
- **I** = **I**nhabitants (around us)
- **T** = **T**radition (or societal norms)
- **A** = **A**cts (or laws)
- **T** = **T**eaching (we receive)

Chapter Fourteen

Home

Most children spend about six hours a day in school. The rest of the time is spent at home and within the community. We as humans are social animals. Our lifestyle is shaped by our interaction with others in the environment. Our family is the immediate environment which influences most of our early childhood development. The home influences child development through values, safety, learning of developmental skills and socialisation.

Children pick up good and bad values by observing their parents and other siblings. Values such as respect, love, empathy and the importance placed on healthy lifestyles are all picked up by children. The family provides immediate emotional and physical safety for children. They learn development skills such as language, movement and reasoning skills which are necessary for optimal growth and development; they observe the physical activity of their parents and the emphasis they place on exercise. Finally, children learn from their family members how to interact with others. Spending quality time together as a family watching TV, having meals or going out together helps develop the child's social skills which are important for survival later in life.

Children pick up good and bad values by observing their parents and their siblings

The family is therefore at the centre of lifestyle development. Families should be engaged in all interventions that seek to modify lifestyle in childhood and the teenage years.

Area (where we live)

The area or community where we live has a major role in our lifestyle. Take identical twins and put them in two different communities. In one community, there are parks for sports where almost everyone goes regularly to exercise, there are cycle tracks and most people go to work using bikes, there is a lot healthy food and almost everyone eats healthily. In the other community, there are no parks, no bike lanes, people are too busy to use bikes, healthy foods are very expensive and most people don't care about the healthiness of the food they eat. It's almost certain that the twin growing up in the first community will adopt a healthy lifestyle compared with the one growing up in the second community.

Lifestyle interventions should take into account the area where we live

In other words, our lifestyle is heavily influenced by where we reside. Lifestyle interventions should take this into account. How do you expect an individual to eat healthily if the society around them is not growing healthy food or if the healthy food is unaffordable?

With globalisation today, the world has become a small village. We are influenced now by areas that are apparently far away physically. Social connections have shortened distances. Social distance is now more influential than physical distance.

Businesses (around us)

Our lifestyle is influenced by the businesses around us. Some food companies carefully craft adverts that show the positives and hide the negatives. Some of these adverts target children who may become victims of deceitful and unethical marketing.

Every day we see adverts for refined carbohydrates and, depending on the country, we can find adverts for tobacco and alcohol too. Because a small amount of a vitamin is added to an unhealthy food to 'fortify' it, publicity will focus on the vitamin to distract attention from the noxious effects of the main component(s) of the food.

Chapter Fourteen

Some food companies carefully craft adverts that show the positives and hide the negatives

Technology is driving the culture of sedentary lifestyle. Studies have shown that we spend about 238 minutes per day watching TV. This is equivalent to 77 days a year spent doing this. In addition to TV, an average person spends 324 minutes per day on their smart phone. This is equivalent to 82 days per year on the phone alone. Imagine what the impact on health would be if just a quarter of this time spent on phones or watching TV were spent on exercise.

Inhabitants

'Inhabitants' – that is, the people around us – have a strong influence on our lifestyle. These people could be friends or people we meet or interact with in our communities. Friends influence each other's personal preferences and lifestyles. If you have a friend who likes exercise, there are higher chances that you will eventually join him or her. Friends also influence the way we think about ourselves. If you have a friend who thinks obesity is normal, you may not see your obesity as an issue. If all your friends smoke or drink alcohol, the chances are high that you will end up doing the same.

People we meet and interact with in our everyday life also have an influence on our lifestyle

People we meet and interact with in our everyday life also have an influence on our lifestyle. For example, a colleague at work who successfully loses weight will influence many of their co-workers to do the same. People influence others by appealing to them either emotionally or logically, and thereby convincing them to act in a particular way.

Tradition (or social norms)

We all trust and believe in superstars. We want to be like them. We admire them and their lifestyles. Every society and every community has a superstar, a celebrity, a champion who is admired by the young people. These role models are very powerful in shaping the trend of our culture and what that society considers normal. Inevitably, organisations use these superstars in their advertisements to send a message to the public that their product or service is the gold standard.

Once the new trend has been adopted by most people, others are bound to follow. If you don't, you become the outlier, the abnormal person who risks being rejected by your society. We are social beings and therefore most people feel forced to move with the trend. Only a few 'deviants' have the audacity to go against the trend.

Acts (or laws)

Our lifestyle is also influenced by the laws (or Acts of Parliament in the UK) that govern our actions and the actions of others, including businesses. Governments have the responsibility to develop laws and policies that prevent diseases of public health importance. Currently, we spend 50 times more money treating diseases than on prevention. Urgent action is therefore required from all governments to shift the focus from treatment to prevention. This is not to say that governments should ignore treatment altogether, but prevention is far cheaper; it does not make sense to invest more in treatment which is more expensive.

Despite the fact that deaths from sick fat disease occur mainly in adulthood, exposure to risk factors such as an unhealthy diet, physical inactivity, alcohol misuse and smoking begins in childhood and builds up throughout the life cycle (children, teenagers, adults and the elderly). Government policies and/or laws can influence the home, area, businesses, inhabitants, traditions and teachings. They should span the entire lifecycle and include the four main modifiable risk factors: diet, physical activity, alcohol use and smoking.

Urgent action is required from all governments to shift the focus from treatment to prevention

Teaching

Our lifestyles are all influenced by the teaching or education we receive throughout our lives, from childhood to adulthood. We learn every day, whether in school or out of school. Nutrition education and physical education should both be incorporated in school curricula. Above all, the education we receive out of school, from the internet, our parents, our friends, our co-workers and other influencers, has a much greater impact. Social media is a powerful tool for education, especially among young people.

Health literacy is more important than ever because health is the new wealth

Health literacy is more important than ever given the rising burden of disease. It's one of the most powerful tools that everyone must have. It is all about how to stay healthy because health is the new wealth and there is no wealth without health.

Glossary of terms

Adrenaline	A hormone produced by the adrenal gland. It's responsible for the 'fight or flight' response.
Aerobic exercise	Aerobic exercise (also called cardio) is any physical exercise that causes an increase in heart rate, such as brisk walking, running or cycling.
Alcohol poisoning	A serious life-threatening condition caused by binge drinking or drinking large amounts of alcohol within a short space of time.
Aldosterone	A hormone produced by the adrenal glands. It causes the kidneys to retain sodium and flush out potassium.
Alzheimer's disease	A progressive disease of the nervous system that destroys memory and other mental functions.
Anorexia	Lack of appetite for food. ('Anorexia nervosa' is the psychiatric condition involving self-starvation.)
Antibodies	Proteins produced by the body's immune system to neutralise pathogens such as bacteria and viruses and their toxins (antigens). Antibodies are 'body soldiers'.
Antigen	A toxin or foreign substance that induces the production of antibodies.
Antioxidant	A substance that inhibits or slows down damage to cells caused by free radicals. They are called 'free radical scavengers'.
Autoimmunity	An abnormal situation where the body's immune system attacks the healthy body tissues and cells.

Autophagy	The process by which the body's cells remove or recycle unnecessary or dysfunctional parts.
Balanced diet	A diet that contains different types of foods in quantities and proportions that provide all the nutrients required by the body.
Binge drinking	Taking a large amount of alcohol within a very short space of time or drinking to get drunk.
Blood clotting disorders	A condition characterised by excessive clotting or blood clot formation. It's also called thrombosis or thromboembolism.
Body mass index (BMI)	A measure of body fat. BMI is weight (in kilos) divided by the square of the height (in metres).
Cancer	A disease in which abnormal cells divide uncontrollably and destroy body tissue.
Carbohydrate	Any of a large group of organic compounds found in foods that include sugars and starch.
Cholesterol	A type of fat found in our cells that is the precursor to many hormones. Abnormally high levels are associated with heart disease. Cholesterol is carried through the bloodstream by proteins called 'lipoproteins' of which there are two types: LDL (low density lipoprotein) and HDL (high density lipoprotein). LDL has been called 'bad' cholesterol because high levels have been associated with atherosclerosis and heart disease. There are two types of LDL cholesterol according to the size of the LDL particles: type A (large dense LDL) and type B (small dense LDL). HDL has been called 'good' cholesterol because it carries cholesterol from the body back to the liver and the liver removes it from the body.
Circadian rhythm	A 24-hour internal clock running in the background in our brains that controls sleep and other functions, such as eating.

Glossary of terms

Cortisol	A steroid hormone produced by the adrenal glands. In excess it causes obesity and sick fat disease.
Cytokines	A large category of signaling proteins produced by the immune cells. They regulate body functions and restore order in the internal environment. They are the 'body police'.
Dementia	The symptom of many diseases, including Alzhemier's disease, Lewy body disease and vascular dementia, characterised by memory loss and poor judgement.
Depression	A disease condition characterised by low mood making the person feel sad, angry, lonely, insecure etc, independent of events and circumstances.
Diabetes	A disease characterised by too much sugar in the blood. Type 1 is characterised by insufficient levels of insulin and type 2 by excessive levels of insulin.
Digestive system	The gastrointestinal tract that takes in food, digests it, extracts and absorbs nutrients, and expels the remaining waste as faeces.
Eclampsia	A life-threatening condition where high blood pressure (pre-eclampsia) in pregnancy results in seizures.
Endocrine system	The body system consisting of glands that produced hormones. It's the 'key-worker' system of the body.
Exercise	A planned physical activity designed to maintain physical fitness and wellbeing.
Fat	One of the main body nutrients (along with carbohydrates and proteins) that provide energy and keep the body warm.
Fatty liver disease	Disease caused by the build-up of fat in the liver.
Fibre	Dietary material containing substances such as cellulose, lignin and pectin that are resistant to the action of digestive enzymes.

Foetal alcohol spectrum disorder	A name for various health, behaviour and learning problems that can affect babies if their mother drinks alcohol in pregnancy.
Foetal alcohol syndrome	A type of foetal alcohol spectrum disorder where the baby presents with brain damage and growth problems.
Free fatty acids (FFAs)	The form in which fats leave the cell and are transported for use in another part of the body. The fatty acids are free, unbound to protein.
Gestational diabetes	A condition where the blood sugar levels become chronically high during pregnancy.
Gestational hypertension	High blood pressure that develops in women during pregnancy. If it's accompanied by protein in the urine, it's called pre-eclampsia.
Ghrelin	Ghrelin or the hunger hormone is produced by the stomach when the body needs energy. Ghrelin enters the 'feeding centre' of the brain (in the hypothalamus) and activates hunger.
Glucagon	A hormone produced by the pancreas. It converts glycogen in the muscles and liver to sugar.
Glycogen	Long chains of sugar (a cluster of sugar) stored in the liver and muscles.
Heart attack	Life-threatening condition caused by blockage of blood flow to the heart, often by a blood clot.
Heart disease	Also called coronary heart disease, this is a life-threatening condition characterised by the build up of plaque in coronary arteries limiting blood flow to the heart.
High blood pressure	A condition in which the force of blood against the artery walls is too high.
Hormone	Hormones are chemical messengers secreted into the blood. I call them 'key workers' because they perform the essential body functions.

Glossary of terms

Hormone replacement therapy (HRT) — HRT is the treatment of symptoms of menopause and bone loss after menopause with oestrogen or combined oestrogen and progestogen.

Hypertension — Another name for high blood pressure.

Immune system — The body's defence system that produces antibodies, cytokines, specialised defence cells, etc.

Insulin — A hormone produced by the pancreas. It reduces blood sugar levels.

Insulin resistance — A situation where the body's cells respond less and less to insulin, so insulin is unable to do its job of delivering sugar into the cells for energy and the pancreas produces increasing amounts of insulin to mitigate the problem.

Intermittent fasting — An eating pattern consisting of cycles with periods of abstinence from food and periods of eating.

Ketosis — The process whereby fats are broken down into ketones and energy is released for the body.

Leptin — A hormone produced by fatty tissues that regulates satiety. Leptin, the satiety hormone, reduces hunger by stimulating the 'satiety centre' of the brain (in the hypothalamus).

Metabolic syndrome — A cluster of diseases consisting of a combination of obesity, high blood pressure, high cholesterol and (eventually) type 2 diabetes. It's also called sick fat disease.

Multiple sclerosis — An autoimmune disease where the body's immune or defence system eats away the protective covering of nerves. It can lead to loss of vision, pain, loss of coordination and fatigue.

Neoplasm — Another name for cancer.

Nervous system — A highly complex body system made up of a network of nerves that ensure electrical signaling between different parts of the body.

Neuro-degenerative disorders	Disease conditions that involve the death or decay of certain parts of the brain. They include Parkinson's disease and Alzheimer's disease.
Obesity	A disorder characterised by excess body fat that increases the risk of health problems.
Oxidative stress	The process by which oxygen free radicals injure body tissues and cells. This occurs when there are not enough antioxidants to neutralise the free radicals.
Oxygen free radicals	Usually called 'free radicals', oxygen free radicals are unstable molecules or substances produced by the body in response to environmental and other pressures. They damage body cells.
Parkinson's disease	A disease of the brain characterised by slow movement, tremors, loss of balance and stiffness.
Physical activity	Bodily movement produced by skeletal muscles that requires expenditure of energy. Exercise is a type of physical activity that is planned specifically for fitness and health.
Pituitary–adrenal axis	Also called the hypothalamic–pituitary–adrenal axis. It's a system that plays a key part in the body's response to stress.
Post-traumatic stress disorder (PTSD)	A health condition due to failure to recover after experiencing or witnessing a terrifying event. It may last for months or years with triggers that bring back the memories of the trauma.
Pre-eclampsia	A pregnancy complication characterised by high blood pressure and protein in the urine.
Processed food	Foods that have been altered in some way during preparation, by freezing, sweetening, canning, baking or drying. What makes processing bad is the removal of fibre or the adding of sugar, salt or fat and the denaturing of carbs, fats and proteins as a result of high temperatures and other processes.

Glossary of terms

Proteins	An essential nutrient that forms part of a balanced diet and is made up of amino acids. They provide the essential building blocks of body tissue and can serve as a fuel source. The essential amino acids are those which cannot be made by the body and therefore must come from food.
Renin–angiotensin system	The hormone system that regulates sodium absorption by the kidneys and, thereby, blood pressure.
Rheumatoid arthritis	A chronic inflammatory disorder caused by autoimmunity that can affect multiple joints.
Schizophrenia	A mental disease characterised by thoughts, feelings and behaviours that seem out of touch with reality.
Sick fat disease	A cluster of symptoms consisting of a combination of obesity, high blood pressure, high cholesterol and type 2 diabetes. It's also called metabolic syndrome.
Slipped disc	Also called disc prolapse, this is a condition where the soft tissue cushion between the bones in the spine pushes out through a crack in the tougher external casing.
Stress	A discomfort caused by any event or thought that makes one feel frustrated, angry, nervous or unable to cope. Stress is the body's way of reacting to a challenge or demand.
Stroke	A life-threatening condition where blood supply to the brain is cut off.
Sympathetic nervous system	One of the two main divisions of the autonomic nervous system (the other being the parasympathetic nervous system) that is responsible for rapid involuntary response to dangerous or stressful situations among other things. The autonomic nervous system is a control system that acts largely unconsciously and regulates bodily functions, such as the heart rate, digestion, respiratory rate, pupillary response in the eye, urination, and sexual arousal.

Thrombosis	The formation of a blood clot in a blood vessel.
Type 1 diabetes	Diabetes caused by lack of insulin, the hormone that keeps blood sugar at a healthy level by helping cells to take in sugar to be used for energy.
Type 2 diabetes	Diabetes caused by insulin resistance, a situation where the body cells become progressively insensitive to insulin.
Waist-to-hip ratio (WHR)	Waist circumference divided by the hip circumference. WHR measures abdominal fat and therefore is more reliable than BMI in predicting the likelihood of a person falling sick.
White-coat hypertension	A situation where some people exhibit blood pressure above the normal range in clinical settings, although they do not show high blood pressure when elsewhere.

References

1. Shi J, Yang Z, Niu Y, Zhang W, et al. Large thigh circumference is associated with lower blood pressure in overweight and obese individuals: a community-based study. *Endocr Connect* 2020; 9(4): 271–278.
2. Ravnskov U, de Lorgeril M, Diamond DM, Hama R, Hamazaki T, Hammarskjöld B, McCully KS. LDL-C does not cause cardiovascular disease: a comprehensive review of the current literature. *Expert Review of Clinical Pharmacology* 2018; 11(10): 959–970.
3. Tsoupras A, Lordan R, Zabetakis I. Inflammation, not cholesterol, is a cause of chronic disease. *Nutrients* 2018; 10(5): 604.
4. Wang N, Fulcher J, Abeysuriya N, Park L, Kumar S, Di Tanna GL, Lal S. Intensive LDL cholesterol-lowering treatment beyond current recommendations for the prevention of major vascular events: a systematic review and meta-analysis of randomised trials including 327 037 participants. *Lancet Diabetes & Endocrinology* 2020; 8(1): 36–49.
5. Calling S, Johansson SE, Wolff M, Sundquist J, Sundquist K. The ratio of total cholesterol to high density lipoprotein cholesterol and myocardial infarction in Women's health in the Lund area (WHILA): a 17-year follow-up cohort study. *BMC Cardiovascular Disorders* 2019; 19(1): 239.
6. Vitaliano PP, Scanlan JM, Zhang J, Savage MV, Hirsch IB, Siegler IC. A path model of chronic stress, the metabolic syndrome, and coronary heart disease. *PsychosomaticMmedicine* 2002; 64(3): 418–435.
7. Neel JV. Diabetes Mellitus: A "Thrifty" Genotype Rendered Detrimental by "Progress"? *Am J Hum Genet* 1962; 14(4): 353–362.

8. Siri-Tarino PW, Sun Q, Hu FB, Krauss RM. Meta-analysis of prospective cohort studies evaluating the association of saturated fat with cardiovascular disease. *American Journal of Clinical Nutrition* 2010; 91(3): 535–546.
9. Hooper L, Martin N, Jimoh OF, Kirk C, Foster E, Abdelhamid AS. Reduction in saturated fat intake for cardiovascular disease. *Cochrane Database of Systematic Reviews* 2020; 5: CD011737. DOI: 10.1002/14651858.CD011737.pub2.
10. Hu FB, Stampfer MJ, Manson JE, et al. Dietary saturated fats and their food sources in relation to the risk of coronary heart disease in women. *Am J Clin Nutr* 1999; 70: 1001–1008.
11. Simopoulos AP. The importance of the omega-6/omega-3 fatty acid ratio in cardiovascular disease and other chronic diseases. *Experimental Biology and Medicine* 2008; 233(6): 674–688.
12. Xing J, Chen JD. Alterations of gastrointestinal motility in obesity. *Obesity Research* 2004; 12(11): 1723–1732.
13. NHS. Overweight and Obesity Prevalence. Accessed on 21 December 2020 from: https://digital.nhs.uk/data-and-information/publications/statistical/statistics-on-obesity-physical-activity-and-diet/england-2020/part-3-adult-obesity-copy
14. DiStefano JK, Shaibi GQ. The relationship between excessive dietary fructose consumption and paediatric fatty liver disease. *Pediatric Obesity* 2020; e12759.
14a. Kongnyuy EJ, Norman RJ, Flight IHK, Rees MC. Oestrogen and progestogen hormone replacement therapy for peri-menopausal and post-menopausal women: weight and body fat distribution. *Cochrane Database of Systematic Reviews* 1999; 3: CD001018. DOI: 10.1002/14651858.CD001018.
15. Vasselli JR, Scarpace PJ, Harris RBS, Banks WA. Dietary Components in the Development of Leptin Resistance. *Adv Nutr* 2013; 4(2): 164–175.
16. Poti JM, Braga B, Qin B. Ultra-processed Food Intake and Obesity: What Really Matters for Health – Processing or Nutrient Content? *Curr Obes Rep* 2017; 6(4): 420–431.
17. Nolen-Hoeksema S. Bulimia Nervosa In: *Abnormal Psychology* 6th edition. Mcgraw-Hill Education: New York; 2014: 344.
18. Rynders CA, Thomas EA, Zaman A, Pan Z, Catenacci VA, Melanson EL. Effectiveness of Intermittent Fasting and Time-Restricted

References

Feeding Compared to Continuous Energy Restriction for Weight Loss. *Nutrients* 2019; 11(10): 2442.
19. Lean ME, Leslie WS, Barnes AC, et al. Primary care-led weight management for remission of type 2 diabetes (DiRECT): an open-label, cluster-randomised trial. *Lancet* 2018; 391 (10120): 541–551.
20. Ravussin E, Beyl RA, Poggiogalle, E, Hsia DS, Peterson CM. (2019). Early time-restricted feeding reduces appetite and increases fat oxidation but does not affect energy expenditure in humans. *Obesity 2019*; 27(8): 1244–1254.
21. Natalucci G, Riedl S, Gleiss A, Zidek T, Frisch H. Spontaneous 24-h ghrelin secretion pattern in fasting subjects: maintenance of a meal-related pattern. *European Journal of Endocrinology* 2005; 152(6): 845–850.
22. Sutton EF, Beyl R, Early KS, Cefalu WT, Ravussin E, Peterson CM. Early time-restricted feeding improves insulin sensitivity, blood pressure, and oxidative stress even without weight loss in men with prediabetes. *Cell metabolism 2018*; 27(6): 1212–1221.
23. de Cabo R, Mattson MP. Effects of intermittent fasting on health, aging, and disease. *New England Journal of Medicine* 2019; 381(26): 2541–2551.
24. Longo VD, Mattson MP. Fasting: molecular mechanisms and clinical applications. *Cell Metabolism* 2014; 19(2): 181–192.
25. Brandhorst S, Choi IY, Wei M, Cheng CW, Sedrakyan S, Navarrete G, Di Biase S. A periodic diet that mimics fasting promotes multi-system regeneration, enhanced cognitive performance, and healthspan. *Cell Metabolism* 2015; 22(1): 86–99.
26. de Cabo R, Mattson MP. Effects of intermittent fasting on health, aging, and disease. *New England Journal of Medicine* 2019; 381(26): 2541–2551.
27. Superko HR, Pendyala L, Williams PT, Momary KM, King III SB, Garrett BC. High-density lipoprotein subclasses and their relationship to cardiovascular disease. *Journal of Clinical Lipidology* 2012; 6(6): 496–523.
28. Lean ME, Leslie WS, Barnes AC, Brosnahan N, Thom G, McCombie, L, Rodrigues AM. Primary care-led weight management for remission of type 2 diabetes (DiRECT): an open-label, cluster-randomised trial. *Lancet* 2018; 391(10120): 541–551
29. Wilcox G. Insulin and insulin resistance. *Clinical Biochemist Reviews* 2005; 26(2): 19.

30. Muoio DM, Newgard CB. Molecular and metabolic mechanisms of insulin resistance and β-cell failure in type 2 diabetes. *Nature Reviews Molecular Cell Biology* 2008; 9(3): 193–205.
31. Samuel VT, Shulman GI. Mechanisms for insulin resistance: common threads and missing links. *Cell* 2012; 148(5): 852–871.
32. Han HS, Kang G, Kim JS, Choi BH, Koo SH. Regulation of glucose metabolism from a liver-centric perspective. *Experimental & Molecular Medicine* 2016; 48(3): e218–e218.
33. Prasad KN, Bondy SC. Dietary fibers and their fermented short-chain fatty acids in prevention of human diseases. *Bioactive Carbohydrates and Dietary Fibre* 2019; 17: 100170.
34. McRae MP. The benefits of dietary fiber intake on reducing the risk of cancer: an umbrella review of meta-analyses. *Journal of Chiropractic Medicine* 2018; 17(2): 90–96.
35. Kaczmarczyk MM, Miller MJ, Freund GG. The health benefits of dietary fiber: beyond the usual suspects of type 2 diabetes mellitus, cardiovascular disease and colon cancer. *Metabolism* 2012; 61(8): 1058–1066.
36. Baliunas DO, Taylor BJ, Irving H, Roerecke M, Patra J, Mohapatra S, Rehm J. Alcohol as a risk factor for type 2 diabetes: a systematic review and meta-analysis. *Diabetes Care* 2009; 32(11): 2123–2132.
37. Rehm J. The risks associated with alcohol use and alcoholism. *Alcohol Research & Health* 2011; 34(2): 135.
38. Xie XT, Liu Q, Wu J, Wakui M. Impact of cigarette smoking in type 2 diabetes development. *Acta Pharmacologica Sinica* 2009; 30(6): 784–787.
38a. Rosenthal T. Seasonal variations in blood pressure. *American Journal of Geriatric Cardiology* 2004; 13(5): 267–272.
39. Fortenberry K, Ricks J, Kovach FE. How much does weight loss affect hypertension?. *Journal of Family Practice* 2013; 62(5): 258–259.
40. Wood AM, Kaptoge S, Butterworth AS, Willeit P, Warnakula S, Bolton T, Bell S. Risk thresholds for alcohol consumption: combined analysis of individual-participant data for 599 912 current drinkers in 83 prospective studies. *Lancet* 2018; 391(10129): 1513–1523.
41. Mathews MJ, Liebenberg L, Mathews EH. The mechanism by which moderate alcohol consumption influences coronary heart disease. *Nutrition Journal* 2015; 14(1): 33.

References

42. Silveri MM. Adolescent brain development and underage drinking in the United States: identifying risks of alcohol use in college populations. *Harvard Review of Psychiatry* 2012; 20(4): 189–200.
43. Chiolero A, Faeh D, Paccaud F, Cornuz J. Consequences of smoking for body weight, body fat distribution, and insulin resistance. *American Journal of Clinical Nutrition* 2008; 87(4): 801–809.
44. Pittilo M. Cigarette smoking, endothelial injury and cardiovascular disease. *International Journal of Experimental Pathology* 2000; 81(4): 219–230.
45. Omvik P. How smoking affects blood pressure. *Blood Pressure* 1996; 5(2): 71–77.
46. Benowitz NL, Burbank AD. Cardiovascular toxicity of nicotine: implications for electronic cigarette use. *Trends in Cardiovascular Medicine* 2016; 26(6): 515–523.
47. Karvonen M, Orma E, Keys A, Fidanza F, Brozek J, Cigarette smoking, serum cholesterol, blood pressure, and body fatness observations in Finland. *Lancet* 1959; 273(7071): 492–494.
48. Leone A. How and why chemicals from tobacco smoke can induce a rise in blood pressure. *World J Pharmacol* 2012; 1(1): 10–20.
49. Gepner AD, Piper ME, Johnson HM, Fiore MC, Baker TB, Stein JH. Effects of smoking and smoking cessation on lipids and lipoproteins: outcomes from a randomized clinical trial. *American Heart Journal* 2011; 161(1): 145–151.
50. Campbell SC, Moffatt RJ, Stamford BA. Smoking and smoking cessation—the relationship between cardiovascular disease and lipoprotein metabolism: a review. *Atherosclerosis* 2008; 201(2): 225–235.
51. Zaratin ÁC, Quintão EC, Sposito AC, Nunes VS, Lottenberg AM, Morton RE., de Faria EC. Smoking prevents the intravascular remodeling of high-density lipoprotein particles: implications for reverse cholesterol transport. *Metabolism* 2004; 53(7): 858–862.
52. Bakhru A, Erlinger TP. Smoking cessation and cardiovascular disease risk factors: results from the Third National Health and Nutrition Examination Survey. *PLoS Med* 2005; 2(6): e160.
53. Hunter KA, Garlick PJ, Broom I, Anderson SE, McNurlan MA. Effects of smoking and abstention from smoking on fibrinogen synthesis in humans. *Clinical Science* 2001; 100(4): 459–465.
54. Maddatu J, Anderson-Baucum E, Evans-Molina C. Smoking and the risk of type 2 diabetes. *Translational Research* 2017; 184: 101–107.

55. National Center for Chronic Disease Prevention and Health Promotion (US) Office on Smoking and Health. The Health Consequences of Smoking – 50 Years of Progress: A Report of the Surgeon General. CDC, Atlanta (GA): 2014. PMID: 24455788.
56. Jacob L, Freyn M, Kalder M, Dinas K, Kostev K. Impact of tobacco smoking on the risk of developing 25 different cancers in the UK: a retrospective study of 422,010 patients followed for up to 30 years. *Oncotarget* 2018; 9(25): 17420.
57. Centers for Disease Control and Prevention (US); National Center for Chronic Disease Prevention and Health Promotion (US); Office on Smoking and Health (US). Atlanta (GA): Centers for Disease Control and Prevention (US); 2010.
58. Laborín R. Smoking and chronic obstructive pulmonary disease (COPD). Parallel epidemics of the 21st century. *International Journal of Environmental Research and Public Health* 2009; 6(1): 209–224.
59. McDonnell BP, Regan C. Smoking in pregnancy: pathophysiology of harm and current evidence for monitoring and cessation. *The Obstetrician & Gynaecologist* 2019; 21(3): 169–175.
60. Mazzone P, Tierney W, Hossain, M, Puvenna V, Janigro D, Cucullo L. Pathophysiological impact of cigarette smoke exposure on the cerebrovascular system with a focus on the blood-brain barrier: expanding the awareness of smoking toxicity in an underappreciated area. *International Journal of Environmental Research and Public Health* 2010; 7(12): 4111–4126.
61. Segerstrom SC, Miller GE. Psychological stress and the human immune system: a meta-analytic study of 30 years of inquiry. *Psychological Bulletin* 2004; 130(4): 601.
62. Bremner DJ. Stress and brain atrophy. *CNS & Neurological Disorders – Drug Targets* 2006; 5(5): 503–512.
63. Ranabir S, Reetu K. Stress and hormones. *Indian Journal of Endocrinology and Metabolism* 2011; 15(1): 18.
64. Lee MJ, Pramyothin P, Karastergiou K, Fried SK. Deconstructing the roles of glucocorticoids in adipose tissue biology and the development of central obesity. *Biochimica et Biophysica Acta (BBA) - Molecular Basis of Disease* 2014; 1842(3): 473–481.
65. Kuo T, McQueen A, Chen TC, Wang JC. Regulation of glucose homeostasis by glucocorticoids. In: *Glucocorticoid Signaling.* Springer: New York, NY; 2015: 99–126.

References

66. Muoio DM, Newgard CB. Molecular and metabolic mechanisms of insulin resistance and β-cell failure in type 2 diabetes. *Nature Reviews Molecular Cell Biology* 2008; 9(3): 193–205.
67. CDC (2012). Lifestyle Coach Facilitator Guide: Post-Core. www.cdc.gov/diabetes/prevention/pdf/PostCurriculum_Session1.pdf. (accessed 20 December 2020).
68. Nystoriak MA, Bhatnagar A. Cardiovascular effects and benefits of exercise. *Frontiers in Cardiovascular Medicine* 2018; 5: 135.
69. Golbidi S, Laher I. Exercise and the aging endothelium. *Journal of Diabetes Research* 2013; 2013: 789607.
70. Laufs U, Werner N, Link A, Endres M, Wassmann S, Jürgens K, Nickenig G. Physical training increases endothelial progenitor cells, inhibits neointima formation, and enhances angiogenesis. *Circulation* 2004; 109(2): 220–226.

Index

abdominal (apple-shaped; upper body; visceral) obesity, 21–22, 51–52, 161, 162
    main causes, 27
    smoking and, 130–131
    stress and, 152
    waist to hip circumference as measure of, 151, 162
acceptance from friends/family, 170–171
ACE inhibitor, 8
acts (law), 180–181
adipose tissue *see* fat
adolescents *see* teenagers
adrenal glands, 53, 99, 101, 147, 151
    see also hypothalamic–pituitary–adrenal axis
adrenaline, 101, 132, 134, 136, 146, 148, 151, 152, 153, **183**
advertising, 180
    food, 178
aerobic (cardio) exercise, 17, 93, 103, 108, 110, 163
    pregnancy, 114
age (and ageing)
    endothelial function and, 163–164
    energy requirements related to, 53–54
    exercise levels and, 54, 113–114
    intermittent fasting and, 72–73
    vitamin D and calcium and, 111
    see also babies; children; older adults; teenagers
agricultural societies, 108
alcohol, 94, 119–128
    binge drinking, 120, 121, 122, 127, **184**
    consensus lacking on low risk limit, 126–127
    long-term effects, 123–124
    moderation, 94, 105, 126–127
    poisoning, 121, 122, **183**
    risks outweighing benefits, 121–124
    short-term effects, 122
    sick fat disease and, 27, 123, 124–125
aldosterone, 99, **183**
Alzheimer's disease, 75, 117, 137, 139, **183**
    intermittent fasting and, 75
ambition and motivation, 168
amusement *see* fun and amusement
amygdala, 150, 151
amylin, 84
angiotensin II, 99

Note: bold reference numbers indicate Glossary entries.

annual health checks, 164–165
anorexia, 60, 61
antibodies, 21, 150, **183**
antidiabetic drugs, 84–85
    author's use, 1, 2, 8, 9, 12, 17, 79–80
    metformin, 8, 13, 79, 84–85
antigens, 150, **183**
antihypertensive (blood pressure-reducing) medicines, 101, 103, 163
    author's use, 1, 2, 14–15, 17, 97
    exercise and stopping BP pills, 103, 105
antioxidants, 24, 73, **183**
approval and praise, 172–173
    physical activity, 172–173
    smoking cessation, 142
apps (health), 67, 159, 160, 170
area (where we live), 177–178
arthritis, rheumatoid, 75, 150, **189**
assistance *see* support
asthma and intermittent fasting, 74
atherogenesis, 24
    smoking and, 132, 134
atherosclerosis, 24, 25, 132–134
    smoking and, 132–134, 135
autoimmunity and autoimmune diseases, 75, **183**
    stress and, 149–150
autonomic nervous system, 100, **189**
    see also parasympathetic nervous system; sympathetic nervous system
autophagy, 73, 75, **184**

babies (maternal factors affecting)
    alcohol, 125–126
    diabetes, 94
    smoking, 139–140
balance exercises, 112
basal metabolic rate (BMR), 67, 68
    age-related, 53
beans and pulses, 33, 36–37
beef, 36, 37
behavioural change, 168, 169
    accelerators of, 168
    see also lifestyle
behavioural symptoms of stress, 145
β-cells producing, 84, 94, 135–136
binge drinking, 120, 121, 122, 127, **184**
binge eating disorder, 62
blood–brain barrier and smoking, 140
blood clot (thrombosis), 21, 73, **184**, **190**
    ageing and intermittent fasting and, 73
    smoking and, 135
blood pressure (BP), 97–106, 131–134, 162–164
    ageing and intermittent fasting and, 73
    alcohol and, 124
    author's, and its management, 1–3, 5–8, 14–18, 43, 97–98, 157–158
    diastolic, 99, 108, 143, 163
    drugs reducing *see* antihypertensive medicines
    high *see* hypertension

Note: bold reference numbers indicate Glossary entries.

Index

monitoring, 162–164
smoking and, 131–134
stress and, 154–155
systolic, 98, 105, 108, 143, 163
blood sugar (blood glucose)
dietary fibre and, 90–92
fasting, 6, 13, 131
smoking and, 136
stress and, 153
weight loss and, 89
blood vessel
constriction (vasoconstriction), 23, 132
dilation (vasodilation), 73, 163
endothelium *see* endothelium
body mass index (BMI), 7–8, 50, 51, 52, 93, 161–162, **184**
author's, 7–8
bone health, 111
exercise and, 116
bowel (intestines)
cancer, diet and, 37, 92
fibre and, 91–92
brain (and neurological function)
adverse effects
alcohol, 122, 123, 128
smoking, 138, 139–140
stress, 148, 150–151
positive effects, exercise, 116
see also neurodegenerative disorders
breath, bad, 49, 87
bulimia (nervosa), 61–62
businesses around us, 178–179

cadmium, cigarette smoke, 139
calcium deficiency, 30, 111
calories (intake/consumption), 80–84
excess, 48, 67, 76, 80–84
measuring (and calories burned), 67–68, 160
pregnancy and, 95
reducing/restricting, 13, 38, 45, 49, 57, 59, 63, 69, 72, 74, 78, 87, 92
24-hour intermittent fasting plan, 78
cancer (neoplasms/tumours), 74, **184**
alcohol and, 123
bowel, diet and, 37, 92
exercise and, 116
intermittent fasting and, 74
smoking and, 137, 138
captopril, 99
carbohydrates (and sugars/glucose), 46–47, **184**
as energy source, 46–47
excess consumption/high dietary levels, 20, 21, 47, 48, 52, 59, 80–84, 88, 92
processed/refined, 38–39, 55, 89, 178
reducing intake, 38, 40, 49, 88–89, 92
starchy, 34, 38–39, 40–41, 46, 86, 88
switch from burning carbs to burning fat (for weight loss), 49–50, 58, 69, 72, 74, 86, 93
see also fibre
carbon monoxide, cigarette smoke, 132, 133, 138

cardio exercise *see* aerobic exercise
cardiovascular system (and disease)
    dietary fat and, 35
    smoking and, 131–134
    see also heart disease
children
    energy requirements, 53
    exercise requirements, 114
    fatty liver disease, 52
    poverty and obesity, 28
    school, 177, 181
    see also babies; teenagers
cholesterol, 23–25
    alcohol and, 124–125
    high, 23–25
    smoking and, 134–135
    see also high-density lipoprotein; low-density lipoprotein
chronic obstructive pulmonary disease (COPD), 136, 137–138
circadian rhythm, 70–71, **184**
    weight loss/fasting and, 74, 78, 80–81
clotting *see* blood clot
community, 176, 177, 177–178, 180
COPD (chronic obstructive pulmonary disease), 136, 137–138
coronavirus pandemic, 26, 81
cortisol, 53, 131, 136, 147, 148, 149, 151, 152, 153, **185**
COVID-19 (coronavirus) pandemic, 26, 81
cytokines, 21, 83–84, **185**
    blood pressure and, 23
    inflammatory, 83–84

dairy and alternatives, 34, 37–38
David, Laurie Ellen, 56
Davy, Sir Humphry, 10
dementia, 117, 137, **185**
    vascular, 139
    see also Alzheimer's disease
depression, **185**
diabetes, 25–26, 79–95, **185**
    drug management *see* antidiabetic drugs
    gestational, 94–95, **186**
    myths and misleading claims, 80
    type 1, 26, 80–81, **185**, **190**
    type 2, 20, 26, 79–95, **190**
        alcohol and, 125
        author's, and its management, 1–3, 5–14, 43, 44, 79–80, 157
        intermittent fasting and, 74, 86–89, 92–93, 93
        national food guides and, 40, 41
        practical tips for reversal, 92–94
        smoking and, 135
        stress and, 82, 84, 146, 147, 153
        weight loss and, 79–95
    see also antidiabetic drugs
diastolic blood pressure, 99, 108, 143, 163
diet, 29–40, 50, 58, **183**
    author's, 7, 11, 12–14, 29
    fibre, 39, 55, 56, 90–93, **185**

Note: bold reference numbers indicate Glossary entries.

high carbohydrate, 20, 21, 47, 48, 52, 80–84
intermittent fasting and, 58
pregnancy, 95
quality and quantity, 87–89
in stress management, 155
see also eating; food; nutrient deficiencies
digestive system (gut; gastrointestinal tract), **185**
alcohol effects, 123
stress and, 148, 149
see also bowel; stomach
disc prolapse (slipped disc), 29, **189**
distance covered each day, measuring, 159–160
drinks *see* alcohol; water

eating
deliberate effort to eat healthily, 30–31
excessive *see* overeating
what to eat more and less of, 39–40
see also diet; food
Eatwell Guide (UK), 31, 32, 33, 38, 40, 89
e-cigarettes, 142
eclampsia, 105, **185**
education, 181
eggs, 33, 36–37
elderly *see* older adults
emotional symptoms and disorders caused by stress, 145, 150
prevention/management, 154–155

endocrine system, 151–152, **185**
stress and, 148, 151–152
endoplasmic reticulum stress, 83, 84
endothelium, 140, 163–164
ageing and, 163–164
smoking-related damage, 132–133
energy (and fuel)
carbs as energy source, 46–47
chronic excess consumption of, 82–83
fats as energy source, 46–47
requirements, age-related, 53–54
see also calories
environment, healthy, 175–181
epigenetics, 28
evolutionary history and physical activity, 108–109
exercise, 93–94, 101–103, 105, 107–117, 168–172, **185**
achievability, 169–170
aerobic *see* aerobic exercise
age and levels of, 54, 113–114
ambition, 168
assistance, 170–172
author's, 12–17, 107–108, 167–172
disorders, 60–62
fun with, 170, 171
heart disease and, 109–112, 116
historical perspectives, 108–109
hypertension and, 97–98, 101–103, 105, 114
intensity, 112–113, 167, 171
intermittent fasting and, 89, 93

physical activity and,
    distinction, 115
pregnancy and, 57, 106, 114
recommended amounts, 102
in stress management, 155
support from friends and
    family, 171
tracking progress, 158–160
weight loss and, 56–57, 104
see also physical activity

faeces (stools) and dietary fibre,
    91–92
family
    help from *see* acceptance;
        support
    at home, 177
fasting, 63–78
    ancient tradition, 65–67
    blood sugar, 6, 13, 131
    intermittent *see* intermittent
        fasting
fat (body fat/adipose tissue), 46,
    55, 83, **185**
    as energy source, 46–47
    excess *see* obesity
    switch from carbs to fats (for
        weight loss), 49–50, 58,
        69, 72, 74, 86, 93
    see also lipid
fat (dietary) *see* oils and fat
fatty acids
    free (FFAs), 20–21, 22, 23, 52,
        73, 134, 153, **186**
    omega 3, 33, 35, 36, 37
    omega 6, 33, 36, 37
    omega 9, 35
fatty liver, 47, 52, **185**

females (women)
    alcohol poisoning, 122
    energy/calorie requirements,
        37, 39
        by age, 53–54
    smoking, 131
    waist-to-hip ratio, 162
fibre, 39, 55, 56, 90–93, **185**
fight or flight response, 100, 101,
    124, 146, 151
fish, 33, 37
flexibility exercises, 111–112
foetus
    foetal alcohol spectrum
        disorder and foetal
        alcohol syndrome, 135–
        136, **183**
    smoking and, 139
    see also babies
food
    advertising, 178
    eating *see* eating
    five food groups (daily intake),
        31
    friendly and sickness-causing,
        39–40
    hunting and gathering, 108,
        115
    obesity pandemic and
        national guides on,
        40–41
    plate size, 50, 58, 88
    processed *see* processed food
    quality and quantity, 87–89
    reducing/limiting intake, 48,
        88
    see also intermittent fasting
    see also diet; fasting

Note: bold reference numbers indicate Glossary entries.

Index

FOODS (healthy foods), 31
France, alcohol and heart disease, 121
free fatty acids (FFAs), 20–21, 22, 23, 52, 73, 134, 153, **186**
friends and family, help from *see* acceptance; support and assistance
fruit and vegetables, 30, 32–34, 39, 88
fuel *see* energy
fun and amusement
  exercise, 170, 171
  smoking cessation, 151

gastric ulcers and *H. pylori*, 11
gastrointestinal tract *see* digestive system
genetics, body fat excess, 27–28
gestational diabetes, 94–95, **186**
gestational hypertension, 105, **186**
ghrelin, 54, 55, 71, 87, 91, **186**
global dimensions, obesity *see* obesity
glucagon, 46, 153, **186**
gluconeogenesis (glucose synthesis), 81, 143
glucose
  blood *see* blood sugar
  dietary *see* carbohydrates
  metabolism, 46, 49, 52, 81, 83, 143
    cortisol effects, 153
glycated haemoglobin, 6–7, 13
glycogen, 46–47, 49, 50, **186**
  breakdown to sugar (glycogenolysis), 153
  exercise and, 89

intermitting fasting and, 58, 69–70, 89
government role/policy, 176, 180–181
growth hormone, 136
  stress and, 148, 151–152
gut *see* digestive system

habitat in which we live, 176–181
haemoglobin, glycated, 6–7, 13
halitosis (bad breath), 49, 87
HDL *see* high-density lipoprotein
health
  alcohol consumption, 122–126
  annual checks, 164–165
  eating healthily, 30–31
  environment and, 175–181
  intermittent fasting and, 72–76
  lifestyle for healthy living, 167–181
  physical inactivity and, 117
  smart phone apps, 67, 159, 160, 170
  smoking and, 136–140
  stress and, 147–153
heart attack, 21, 133, 164, **186**
heart disease, **186**
  alcohol and, 121, 123, 125
  cholesterol and, 24, 25, 121, 125
  stress and, 148
  exercise and, 109–112, 116
  intermittent fasting and, 75, 76
  smoking and, 130, 133, 135
  see also cardiovascular system
Helicobacter pylori and gastric ulcers, 11
high-density lipoprotein (HDL) cholesterol, 25, 75–76

alcohol and, 121, 124–125
intermittent fasting and, 75–76
smoking and, 134, 135
trans fats and, 36
hippocampus, 150–151
Hippocrates, 66
historical perspectives on physical activity and exercise, 108–109
Hofman, Albert, 10
home, 177
hormone(s), 81, 99, 151, **186**
body fat distribution and, 52–53
hunger and satiety regulation, 54–55
stress and, 148, 149, 151–152
see also endocrine system
hormone replacement therapy (HRT), 53, **187**
HRT (hormone replacement therapy), 53, **187**
hunger regulation, 54–55, 71, 87, 91
hunting and gathering food, 108, 115
hydrogenated oils, 36
hypertension (high BP), 23, 97–106, 131–134, **187**
alcohol and, 124, 131–134
author's, and its management, 1–3, 5–8, 14–18, 43, 97–98
drugs for *see* antihypertensive medicines
exercise and, 87–88, 101–103, 104–105, 114
physical inactivity and, 98–101
practical tips, 104–105
in pregnancy, 105–106, **186**

weight loss and, 103–104
white-coat, 5, **190**
hypothalamic–pituitary–adrenal axis (pituitary–adrenal) axis, 145, 147, 148, 151

immune system, 137, 148, **187**
smoking and, 135
stress and, 148, 149–150
industrial workers, 109
inflammation
chronic, obesity-induced, 83–84
intermittent fasting and, 74–75
inhabitants (people around us), 179
insoluble fibre, 55, 90, 91–92
insulin, 25–26, 46, 80–87, **187**
administration in type 2 diabetes, 85
β-cells producing, 84, 94, 135–136
intermittent fasting and, 76
receptors, 81, 83
insulin resistance/insensitivity, 26, 58, 81–84, 86, 86–87, **187**
reducing/treating (improving insulin sensitivity), 86, 93, 94
smoking and, 135
stress and, 83, 84, 153
intensity of exercise, 112–113, 167, 171
intermittent fasting (abstaining from food), 49–50, 58, 63–78, 86–89, 92–93
diabetes type 2 and, 74, 86–89, 92–93, 93

Note: bold reference numbers indicate Glossary entries.

Index

exercise and, 89, 93
health benefits, 72–76
plans, 76–78
weight loss with, 63, 67, 69, 86–89
why it works, 69–71
intestines *see* bowel

joints and stress, 148
see also rheumatoid arthritis

ketones and ketosis, 49, 87, **187**
kidneys, 99
blood pressure and, 23
Krebs' (tricarboxylic acid) cycle, 82, 83

law, 180–181
Lazear, Jesse, 10
LDL *see* low-density lipoprotein
learning,, stress affecting, 150
legislation (law), 180–181
leptin, 54, 55, 91, **187**
lifestyle, 167–181
author's, 2, 7, 175
body fat excess and, 27
change to healthy one, 167–181
environment and, 175–181
pregnancy and blood pressure and, 106
sedentary *see* physical inactivity
sick fat disease and *see* sick fat disease
see also behavioural change
lipid
breakdown (lipolysis), 153
muscle, excess, 83

production, 22, 52
lipoproteins *see* high-density lipoprotein; low-density lipoprotein
liver, 23–24, 25, 52
alcohol and, 122, 123
calorie excess and, 83
fatty, 47, 52, **185**
glycogen and, 46, 86
local environment, 177–178
low-density lipoprotein (LDL)
cholesterol, 24, 25, 52, 75–76, 91, **184**
alcohol and, 121, 124–125
intermittent fasting and, 75–76
smoking and, 134, 135
stress and, 152
trans fats and, 36
lunch, skipping, 13, 16, 17, 18, 50, 64–65, 76, 78
lung disease and smoking, 137–138
lung cancer, 137

males (men)
alcohol poisoning, 122
energy/calorie requirements, 37, 39
by age, 53–54
smoking, 131
waist-to-hip ratio, 162
Marshall, Barry, 10
meat, 37
medical fasting, 66–67
mental illness and alcohol, 124
metabolic syndrome *see* sick fat disease
metformin, 8, 13, 79, 84–85

MONICA Project, 121
monounsaturated fat, 35
motivation and ambition, 168
multiple sclerosis, 75, 139, **187**
  intermittent fasting and, 74
Murphy's Law, 144–145
muscle
  exercise and, 116
  glycogen storage, 46
  lipid excess, 83
  stress and, 148
music
  in exercise, 170
  in stress management, 155
Myplate, 40

national food guides and obesity pandemic, 40–41
Neel, James, 28
neoplasms *see* cancer
nervous system, **187**
  autonomic *see* autonomic nervous system; parasympathetic nervous system; sympathetic nervous system
  stress and, 150–151
  sympathetic, 100–101, 146–147, **190**
neurodegenerative disorders, **188**
  intermittent fasting and, 75
neurological function *see* brain
Newton, Sir Isaac, 10
nicotine, 131, 132, 134, 135, 136, 139, 140
  replacement therapy, 141, 142
nitric oxide, 132, 163–164

nomadic societies, 108, 109
nut(s), 37
nutrient deficiencies, 29
  ageing and, 111
  alcohol and, 123
  calcium, 30, 111
  vitamin D, 111
  see also diet

obesity (overweight; excess body fat), 40–41, 43–62, **188**
  ageing and intermittent fasting and, 74
  alcohol and, 124
  BMI and, 50, 161
  chronic inflammation induced by, 83–84
  exercise and, 56, 116
  genetic factors, 28
  global pandemic of, 44
  national food guides and, 40–41
  lower body (pear-shaped), 21–22, 51, 152, 161, 162
  media myths, 45
  overeating and, 47–48
  upper body *see* abdominal obesity
obsessive–compulsive disorder (OCD), 60–61
oestrogen, 52, 53, 131, 152
oils and fat (dietary), 33, 34–36
  excess intake, 84
  saturated, 34–35, 35, 37, 38, 121
  trans fats, 36
  unsaturated *see* unsaturated fat
older adults/elderly
  energy requirements, 54

Note: bold reference numbers indicate Glossary entries.

Index

exercise recommendations, 114
see also age
omega 3 fatty acids, 33, 35, 36, 37
omega 6 fatty acids, 33, 36, 37
omega 9 fatty acids, 35
optimism, 155
orthorexia, 60–61
overeating (excess eating/food intake), 21–22, 41, 45, 47–48
    carbohydrates/sugars, 38, 47, 52, 80–84
    obesity and, 47–48
    processed food and, 55–56
    see also calories
overweight *see* obesity
oxidative stress, 72, **188**
    obesity and, 83
    smoking and, 139, 140
oxygen free radicals (free radicals), 72–73, 132, **188**

pancreas, 25–26, 46, 81
    alcohol effects, 123
    β-cells, 84, 94, 135–136
    regeneration, 74, 78
parasympathetic nervous system, 100, **189**
Parkinson's disease, 72, 75, **188**
people around us (inhabitants), 179
physical activity, 54, 56, 116, **188**
    assistance, 170–172
    exercise and, distinction, 115
    key points, 108
    monitoring, 158–160
    throughout the day, 107–108, 115
    see also exercise

physical inactivity (sedentary lifestyle)
    health cost, 115–117
    hypertension and, 98–101
physical symptoms of stress, 145
pituitary–adrenal axis (PAA), 145, 147, 148, 151
poisonous chemicals *see* toxic/poisonous chemicals
polyunsaturated fat, 34, 35, 36
post-traumatic stress disorder (PTSD), 147, **188**
potassium, 23, 99
praise *see* approval and praise
prayer, 156
pre-eclampsia, 94, **185**, **186**, **188**
pre-frontal cortex, 150, 151
pregnancy
    alcohol effects, 123, 125–126
    diabetes (gestational diabetes), 94–95, **186**
    diet in, 39
    exercise and, 57, 106, 114
    fasting and, 71
    hypertension (incl. gestational hypertension), 106, **186**
    smoking and, 136, 138–139
processed (refined) food, 55–56, 89, 91, **188**
    carbohydrates, 38–39, 55, 89, 178
    meat, 37
    overeating and, 55–56
proteins, 36–37, **189**
    dietary sources, 33, 36–37
protest, fasting as form of, 66

psychiatric (mental) illness and alcohol, 124
PTSD (post-traumatic stress disorder), 147, **188**
pulses and beans, 33, 36–37
purging, 61, 62

ramipril, 8, 15, 16, 17, 99
refined food *see* processed food
religious purposes, fasting, 65–66
  see also prayer
renin–angiotensin system (RAS), 99, 100
  exercise and, 102
resistance (strength) training, 93–94, 110–111
rheumatoid arthritis, 75, 150, **189**
Risk Threshold Study, 121

salt intake, 6, 7, 23, 56
satiety regulation, 55, 91
saturated fat, 34–35, 35, 37, 38, 121
schizophrenia, 124, **189**
school, 177, 181
sedentary lifestyle *see* physical inactivity
self-experimentation, 10–11
sex hormones, 52–54, 131, 152
sick fat disease (metabolic syndrome), 19–28, **187, 189**
  abdominal fat and, 50–53
  alcohol and, 27, 123, 124–125
  author's experience, 176
  hypertension and, 99
  lifestyle and, 22
    exercise and physical activity/inactivity, 115–116, 117

prevention, 26–28
SAFEST acronym in management of, 104–105
smoking and, 27, 130–136
stress and, 27, 145–147, 145–147, 148, 152–154
sympathetic nervous system and, 101, 145–147
slipped disc, 29, **189**
smart phones, 179
  health apps, 67, 159, 160, 170
smoking, 94, 129–142
  author's friend, 129–130
  health costs, 136–140
  never starting, 140–141
  passive, 133–134, 137, 138
  quitting, 94, 105, 141–142
  sick fat diseases and, 27, 130–136
snacks, stopping, 13, 16, 17, 58, 64, 65, 76, 78
social norms, 180
social support *see* support
sodium and blood pressure, 23, 73, 99
solidarity, fasting as form of, 66
soluble fibre, 55, 90, 91, 92
speedometer, 159, 160
standing work station, 115
starchy carbohydrates, 34, 38–39, 40–41, 46, 86, 88
steps per day (and tracking it), 158–159, 169–170
stomach
  shrinking with intermittent fasting, 50, 58, 71, 88
  ulcers and *H. pylori*, 11
stools and dietary fibre, 91–92

Note: bold reference numbers indicate Glossary entries.

Index

strength training, 93–94, 110–111
stress, 143–150, **189**
    acute, 147, 151
    ageing and intermittent fasting and, 73
    author's, 143–144
    chronic, 147, 148, 149–150, 152–153, 154
    diabetes (or insulin resistance) and, 82, 84, 146, 147, 153
    health costs, 147–153
    management, 94, 105, 153–156
    sick fat diseases and, 27, 145–147
    see also oxidative stress
stress stoppers, 154
stretching exercises, 111–112
stroke, 189
sucrose, 52
sugar *see* blood sugar; carbohydrates
support and assistance (friends and family), 6, 170–172
    physical activity, 170–172
    stopping smoking, 142
    stress management, 155
sympathetic nervous system, 100–101, 146–147, **189**
    alcohol and, 124
    exercise and, 102
    sick fat disease and, 101, 145–147
    stress and, 145, 146–147, 148, 150, 151, 152, 153
systolic blood pressure, 98, 105, 108, 143, 163

tar, cigarette smoke, 138–139

teaching, 181
technology, 179
    smart phones *see* smart phones
teenagers/adolescents/young adults
    alcohol consumption, 128
    author's experience, 175
    energy requirements, 53, 54
    fatty liver disease, 52
testosterone, 52, 131, 152
thrifty genotype hypothesis, 28
thrombosis *see* blood clot
thyroid hormones, 151
toxic/poisonous chemicals
    alcohol poisoning, 121, 122, **183**
    binding to insoluble fibre, 90
    smoking, 136, 137, 138, 139, 140, 142
tradition, 180
trans fats, 36
trials (author's)
    blood pressure reduction, 2–3, 5, 14–18, 157
    diabetes reversal, 2–3, 5, 8–14, 157
tricarboxylic acid (Krebs') cycle, 82, 83
tumours *see* cancer
20/80 rule
    first, 57, 104
    second, 57, 104
    third, 104

UK *see* United Kingdom
ulcers, gastric, and *H. pylori*, 11
United Kingdom (UK)
    alcohol low risk limits, 127

coronavirus in, 81
Eatwell Guide, 31, 32, 33, 38, 40, 89
health checks with GP, 165
sick fat disease, 176
United States (USA)
  alcohol low risk limits, 127
  Myplate, 40
  smoking and COPD-related deaths, 138
unsaturated fat (dietary), 35, 37
  monounsaturated fat, 35
  polyunsaturated fat, 34, 35, 36
US *see* United States

vaping (e-cigarettes), 142
vascular dementia, 139
vasoconstriction (blood vessel constriction), 23, 132
vasodilation (blood vessel dilation), 73, 163
vegetables and fruit, 30, 32–34, 39, 88
vitamin D deficiency, 111

waist-to-hip ratio (WHR), 131, 160, 162–163, **190**

walking, 11, 16–17
  steps per day (and tracking number), 158–159, 169–170
water (drinking), 38, 50, 59
  fasting and, 59, 77
weight loss, 45–62, 79–95, 104, 161
  ABCDE of, 58–60
  author's, 12–14, 44, 167
  blood sugar and, 89
  diabetes type 2 and, 79–95
  exercise and, 56–57, 103–104
  hypertension and, 103–104
  with intermittent fasting, 63, 67, 69, 86–89
  key points for those wanting to lose weight, 45
  monitoring, 161
  switch from burning carbs to burning fats for, 49–50, 58, 69, 72, 74, 86, 93
white-coat hypertension, 5, **190**
women *see* females

yoga, 156
young people *see* children; teenagers

Also from Hammersmith Health Books

Could it be Insulin Resistance?

By Hanna Purdy

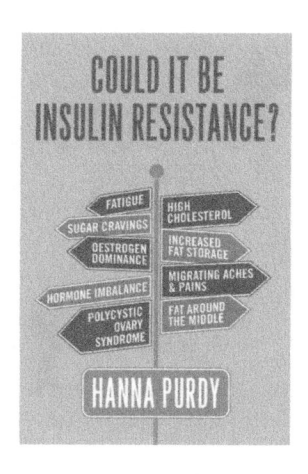

Do you have high cholesterol? And/or high blood pressure? Perhaps a diagnosis of fatty liver? Are you tired all the time? Do you crave sweet snacks? Are your hormones in turmoil? Do you have a bit too much fat around your middle? Your doctor may have tested you for type 2 diabetes and found this is not a problem… yet. But you almost certainly already have its precursor – insulin resistance. Nurse Practitioner Hanna Purdy shares her long experience in Public Health Nursing, as well as with improving her own family's health, to present this practical, evidence-based guide to what 'insulin resistance' means, what causes it and what to do about it, including how to start a ketogenic/low-carb diet, with the emphasis on the quality of food eaten and the impact good food can have on the body and mind.

Also from Hammersmith Health Books

Conquer Type 2 Diabetes

How a fat, middle-aged man lost 31 kilos and reversed his type 2 diabetes

By Richard Shaw

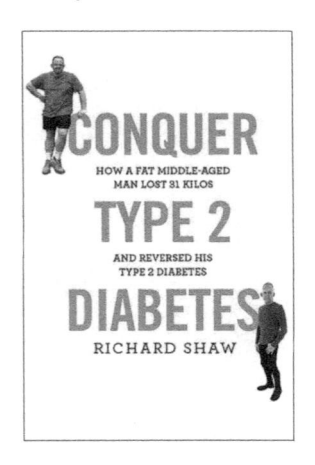

Type-2 diabetes doesn't have to be a lifelong condition; for many people, especially those who have been recently diagnosed, it's possible to reverse the symptoms of this malignant disease. But how can that be done? In 2017 the author, inspired by results obtained from research done at Newcastle University, UK, decided to try and kick the disease by following a carefully structured, low-carb, whole-food diet and starting a modest exercise regime. Conquer Type 2 Diabetes describes what he did to lose 31 kilos and all his diabetes signs and symptoms. It explains how he managed carbs, calories, sugars and weight loss, plus the light exercise regime he adopted to strengthen his chances. In so doing he answers the question so many people have been asking him – what did you do to shed an illness that affects more than 400 million people worldwide and is conventionally regarded as incurable and progressive?